Nursing School, NCLEX and Career Transition Success

Cheryl Thompson

Nursing School, NCLEX and Career Transition Success

Think, Learn, Succeed

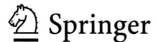

Cheryl Thompson, DNP, RN, PHCNS-BC
Cheryl Thompson Consulting, LLC
Wrightsville, PA, USA

ISBN 978-3-031-85537-5   ISBN 978-3-031-85538-2   (eBook)
https://doi.org/10.1007/978-3-031-85538-2

© The Editor(s) (if applicable) and The Author(s), under exclusive license to Springer Nature
Switzerland AG 2025

This work is subject to copyright. All rights are solely and exclusively licensed by the Publisher,
whether the whole or part of the material is concerned, specifically the rights of translation,
reprinting, reuse of illustrations, recitation, broadcasting, reproduction on microfilms or in any
other physical way, and transmission or information storage and retrieval, electronic adaptation,
computer software, or by similar or dissimilar methodology now known or hereafter developed.
The use of general descriptive names, registered names, trademarks, service marks, etc. in this
publication does not imply, even in the absence of a specific statement, that such names are
exempt from the relevant protective laws and regulations and therefore free for general use.
The publisher, the authors and the editors are safe to assume that the advice and information in
this book are believed to be true and accurate at the date of publication. Neither the publisher nor
the authors or the editors give a warranty, expressed or implied, with respect to the material
contained herein or for any errors or omissions that may have been made. The publisher remains
neutral with regard to jurisdictional claims in published maps and institutional affiliations.

This Springer imprint is published by the registered company Springer Nature Switzerland AG
The registered company address is: Gewerbestrasse 11, 6330 Cham, Switzerland

If disposing of this product, please recycle the paper.

To Tim. A better partner could not be found.

Preface

This book is designed to be a practical, hands-on guide to help you develop skills and strategies to succeed in nursing school, on the National Council of State Boards of Nursing licensing exam (NCLEX®), and in nursing practice.

In recent years clinical nursing practice has changed dramatically. Today's healthcare environment demands more from nurses than ever before. These nursing practice changes have trickled down to nursing education, intensifying the challenges of nursing school.

Whether you're in a practical/vocational, associate, or bachelor's program in this book you will find strategies to:

- Develop effective critical thinking skills
- Optimize your learning and study habits
- Manage stress and maintain a healthy lifestyle
- Prepare effectively for NCLEX
- Transition into your nursing career with confidence and success

Throughout the book, you'll find self-assessment tools, activities, exercises, and real-world examples to help you apply the concepts you're learning. If you're using this book on your own, taking time to complete the activities will enhance your learning. The activities reinforce key concepts and help develop critical thinking skills by applying your learning.

If you're using this book as part of a course, your instructor may incorporate the learning activities as part of your course assignments.

The challenges you face in nursing school are preparing you for the exciting real-world demands of nursing. Embrace the journey, and let this book be your guide to success.

I wish you all the best in your nursing education and future career. The nursing profession will be richer for having you join its ranks.

Wrightsville, PA, USA
November 2024

Cheryl Thompson, DNP, RN, PHCNS-BC

About the Book

This book is structured to support your success throughout your nursing education journey. It is divided into four key parts:

- Part I: Foundation for Thinking and Learning in Nursing School
  - This section introduces you to critical thinking and brain-based learning concepts essential for nursing education. It provides the groundwork for understanding how to optimize your learning process.
- Part II: Toolkit for Nursing School Success
  - Here you'll find practical strategies for managing various aspects of your nursing school experience.
- Part III: NCLEX and Career Planning
  - This part focuses on preparing you for the NCLEX exam and planning your nursing career.
- Part IV: Transition to Nursing Practice
  - The final section supports your move from nursing school to professional practice.

Throughout each chapter, you'll find:

- Self-assessment tools to identify your strengths and areas for improvement
- Activities and exercises to apply concepts you're learning
- Real-world examples and case studies illustrating key points

For Nursing Instructors

This book can serve as a supplementary resource for any nursing course. While the book content serves all nursing students, it is of particular importance for students who will benefit from targeted support for academic success early in their nursing school career.

The self-assessments, activities, and real-world examples throughout this book can be incorporated into your curriculum as assignments, discussion prompts, or group projects. These tools help evaluate student competency, reinforce key concepts, and promote active learning. By integrating these elements into your teaching, you can help students develop essential skills for success in nursing education and practice.

Whether you're a nursing student seeking to excel in your nursing education or an instructor seeking to enhance your teaching resources, this book provides tools and strategies nursing education, NCLEX, and career transition success.

Contents

Part I Foundation for Thinking and Learning in Nursing School

1 Critical Thinking: Lay the Foundation for Thinking
Like a Nurse.   3

2 Brain-Based Learning: Support Critical Thinking
with Brain-Based Learning Strategies   19

3 Neuroplasticity: Adopt a Growth Mindset to Power up
Brain-Based Learning   29

Part II Toolkit for Nursing School Success

4 Manage Your Thinking.   41

5 Manage Your Time   53

6 Manage Your Lifestyle   63

7 Manage Stress   77

8 Manage Your Anxiety and Conquer Test Anxiety   91

9 Using AI to Support Your Learning   103

Part III NCLEX and Career Planning

10 Finding Your Ideal First Nursing Job.   117

11 NCLEX Essentials: From Application to Examination.   129

12 Preparing for NCLEX in Your Final Semester   137

13 Preparing for NCLEX After Graduation   145

Part IV Transition to Nursing Practice

14 From Nursing Student to Nurse: Transitioning
to Nursing Practice   161

About the Author

Cheryl Thompson, DNP, RN, PHCNS-BC brings over four decades of nursing experience to this book. She began her career in ICU and home health nursing before transitioning to academia, where she taught for over 25 years in a Bachelor's of Science in Nursing (BSN) program at York College of Pennsylvania. Dr. Thompson's passion lies in helping nursing students overcome academic challenges and reach their goal of becoming a nurse.

With a keen understanding of the struggles many students face, Dr. Thompson has developed innovative strategies to improve learning outcomes and NCLEX readiness. As the founder of NCLEXRx, she provides coaching for individuals seeking NCLEX success and educational consulting to schools of nursing. Her expertise extends to curriculum development, enhancing student learning outcomes, and implementing effective NCLEX preparation strategies.

Dr. Thompson has authored numerous peer-reviewed publications and presentations on nursing education and student success. This is her second book, following "Overcoming NCLEX Failure: A Guide to Retest Success." Her work continues to empower both students and faculty to achieve their educational goals.

Part I

Foundation for Thinking and Learning in Nursing School

Critical Thinking: Lay the Foundation for Thinking Like a Nurse

1

Education is not the learning of facts, but the training of the mind to think.

—Albert Einstein

1.1 Introduction

As you embark on your journey to become a nurse, you'll quickly discover that nursing is more than memorizing facts and following procedures. It's about developing a keen ability to analyze situations, make informed decisions, and provide compassionate care. This chapter will introduce you to the concept of critical thinking and its crucial role in nursing education and practice. You'll learn how to cultivate this essential skill, which will serve as the foundation for your success in nursing school and throughout your career.

▶ **By the end of this chapter you will be able to:**
1. Define critical thinking in the context of nursing education and practice.
2. Identify the key characteristics of critical thinkers.
3. Understand the relationship between critical thinking, clinical reasoning, and clinical judgment.
4. Apply critical thinking strategies to nursing scenarios.
5. Assess your own critical thinking skills and identify areas for improvement.
6. Recognize the importance of reflection in developing critical thinking abilities.

1.2 Critical Thinking in Nursing

Florence Nightingale, nursing's founder, exemplified critical thinking in nursing (Fig. 1.1). During the Crimean War while working as a nurse in a hospital where the injured received care, she analyzed factors affecting soldier survival rates and connected care conditions to soldiers who lived and died. She then took that information to implement practice changes that improved survival as she strove to understand what factors contributed to survival and what factors contributed to death. This is the basic premise of critical thinking in nursing, understanding "why" and "how" and applying a systematic process of thinking so that understanding can be incorporated into nursing care and practice (Caputi, 2017a).

Building on Nightingale's legacy, modern nursing continues to rely heavily on critical

---

© The Author(s), under exclusive license to Springer Nature Switzerland AG 2025
C. Thompson, *Nursing School, NCLEX and Career Transition Success*,
https://doi.org/10.1007/978-3-031-85538-2_1

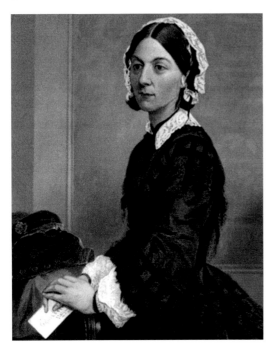

Fig. 1.1 Florence Nightingale in Crimea. (Image created with Artificial Intelligence OpenAI. (2024). Florence Nightingale in Crimea. DALL·E. https://openai.com)

thinking. The work of nurses on the front lines of care is complex, multifaceted, demanding, and fast-paced. Recognizing the crucial role of nursing actions in client outcomes, researchers have sought to understand how nurses think and respond when caring for clients. This research identified "clinical judgment" as the end result of a nurse's critical thinking—nursing action based on client needs.

This research led to models describing "Clinical Judgment" (Dickison et al., 2019). The most widely adopted is Tanner's Clinical Judgment Model (Tanner, 2006), which experts agree best defines the way a nurse thinks about what is happening (clinical decision making) and then provides care based on that thinking (clinical judgment). Your school of nursing is likely to have adopted this model and will teach you about it. Tanner's Clinical Judgment Model is depicted in Fig. 1.2.

Clinical judgment, which is the outcome of nurses' thinking, is rooted in critical thinking. On a diagram, it looks like Fig. 1.3.

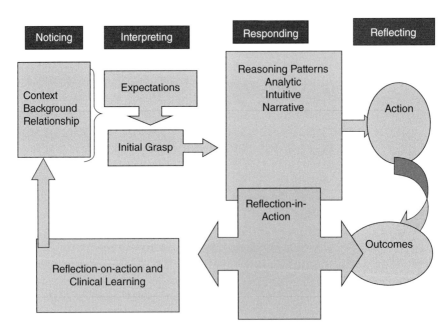

Fig. 1.2 Tanner's Clinical Judgment Model. (Used with Permission)

1.2 Critical Thinking in Nursing

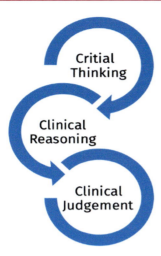

Fig. 1.3 Clinical thinking relationship to clinical reasoning and clinical judgment. (Created by author)

Your critical thinking is the basis for applying your learning to a nursing care scenario (clinical reasoning) and then taking action on that (clinical judgment) and is the foundation for thinking like a nurse. It is also the foundation for nursing school success. Critical thinking will help you learn, understand, remember, and apply information in every setting that is important on your journey to becoming a nurse:

- Class
- Exams
- Simulation
- Clinical
- NCLEX
- Nursing Practice

Your nursing instructors will refer to critical thinking and may assume you know what it means (Caputi & Kavanagh, 2018). But let's not make that assumption here.

1.2.1 Defining Critical Thinking

Critical thinking is the process of analyzing and evaluating information, connecting it to previous knowledge, and applying this understanding to solve problems and innovate in various life situations. While it is embedded in nursing practice, it is a skill you use in your everyday life. It's a versatile skill that helps you make smart choices based on your learning and on previous experience.

You're already using critical thinking skills in many aspects of your life. The purpose of focusing on critical thinking in your nursing education is to enhance these existing abilities and apply them to the process of learning how to think like a nurse. Developing your critical thinking skills will lay the foundation for success in nursing school and in your future nursing practice.

Here's an example of critical thinking in everyday decision-making.

You're preparing to register for next semester's nursing courses. You need to balance your required nursing classes with general education requirements, while also considering your work schedule and family responsibilities. You recently learned about the importance of reviewing class content immediately after each class session to reinforce learning, and you want to incorporate this strategy into your schedule for your nursing courses.

Applying critical thinking to this situation you would:

- **Analyze the situation**
  You review the course catalog, identifying required courses and their prerequisites. You also consider your work schedule, family commitments, and the need for post-class review time. You understand how the course scheduling system works, and why courses are sequenced throughout your nursing program.
- **Gather information**
  You speak with your academic advisor, peer mentors, and upperclassmen about course difficulty and advice. If you have options for different instructors, you may research professors' teaching style and consider which would align best with your learning style.
- **Consider past experiences**
  You reflect on your recent semesters, identifying what contributed to your successes and challenges in retaining information from your nursing classes.
- **Evaluate options**
  You create several possible course combinations, considering factors like course difficulty, scheduling conflicts, and opportunities for immediate post-class review. You look for schedules that allow at least 30 min after each nursing class.
- **Make informed decisions**
  Based on your analysis, you choose a course load that allows time for work and family obligations you can't change. You decide to take nursing courses on Mondays, Wednesdays, and Fridays, with gaps

between classes for study time. You create a weekly schedule that includes class times, work shifts, family commitments, and post-class review periods. You also identify campus locations where you can do your study time and post-class review.

- **Evaluate your decision making**
  You recognize that you may need to adjust your plan as the semester progresses. You're prepared to reassess and make changes if you find certain classes require more review time or if work or family commitments shift.

This everyday example illustrates critical thinking as it pertains to a big decision; selecting a course schedule for an upcoming semester.

You also use critical thinking on a daily basis as you make small decisions about how to plan your day. For example, you prepare for a class that starts at 10 AM. You consider what time you need to leave for class in order to get there on time. Do you need to leave extra time for an errand, to get a snack, to get from the parking lot or bus stop to class? How much extra time do you need based on your previous schedule? Do you need additional time before class to prepare for a class activity or review your notes? Have you arrived late at some point and realized the instructor locks the door? Are there weather conditions that will impact today's timing for getting to class? Why is it important to get to class a few minutes early to prepare yourself for your learning? These are all examples of critical thinking as it relates to your daily decision making.

Completing Pause and Reflect 1.1 Critical Thinking in Action will help you reflect on your own critical thinking.

Pause and Reflect 1.1: Critical Thinking in Action

Consider a decision you made today that involved your having to think through planning and decision making then complete Table 1.1 Critical Thinking in Action.

Completing Table 1.1 helps you see how the process of thinking through decisions contributes to your decision making for the

---

decisions you make as you navigate a day. You also use critical thinking when you make bigger life choices. How did you decide to pursue nursing education? What informed your decision to attend the school you are attending? You could complete Table 1.1 again for these decisions to see how critical thinking contributes to your decision making.

Table 1.1 Critical thinking in action

Decision I made		
Critical thinking step	Critical thinking questions to consider	Your action
Analyze the situation	What did you have to take into consideration as you began your planning? Why are these factors important?	
Gather information	What additional information did you need and how did you determine you needed that information?	
Consider past experience	Why are these experiences relevant? How did they impact the outcome in previous experiences?	
Evaluate options	What alternatives did you have to consider? Why were some options better than others?	
Make informed decision	Based on the thinking thus far, how did you decide to act? Why was this the best decision?	
Evaluate your decision making	Was this the best decision? Why or why not? Is this the same decision you would make in the future given the same circumstance?	

1.2.2 Critical Thinking Mindset for Nursing School Success

In your nursing courses, you'll use critical thinking to deepen your understanding of complex topics, and that understanding will lead to "why" and "how" when you translate that to clinical decisions and clinical judgment. For instance, when learning about a disease you won't just memorize symptoms and treatments. Instead, you'll analyze how symptoms relate to the disease process, evaluate treatment options, and consider how this knowledge applies to nursing care. This critical thinking approach prepares you to answer exam questions effectively and, more importantly, to provide high-quality care to your future clients.

Critical thinking is the foundation for your nursing school success. When you use critical thinking, you enhance your learning in a way that helps you to understand what you have learned (Scheffer & Rubenfeld, 2000). In turn, this understanding helps you to apply your learning throughout nursing school. As depicted in Fig. 1.4, critical thinking will support your success in all aspects of nursing school as you apply your learning in class, in simulation and clinical experiences when you apply clinical decision making to clinical judgment (Lasater, 2007), and on exams, when you apply what you have learned in class. After you graduate from nursing school, you will apply those same critical thinking skills to your NCLEX examination. Critical thinking will continue to be the foundation for your thinking like a nurse in your nursing practice.

In the next section, we will delve deeper into the topic of critical thinking, by looking at the characteristics of critical thinking. Before you read that, complete Self-Assessment 1.1 Critical Thinking Attributes.

Self-Assessment 1.1: Critical Thinking

For each statement in Table 1.2 Critical Thinking Self-Check answer yes or no to see the attributes of critical thinking you embrace.

If you answered "Yes" to most of these questions:

Your curiosity, open-mindedness, and positive attitude toward learning indicate that you

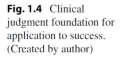

Fig. 1.4 Clinical judgment foundation for application to success. (Created by author)

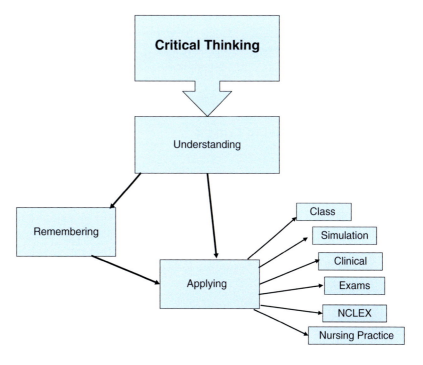

Table 1.2 Clinical thinking self-check

Critical thinking self-check	Yes	No
I enjoy learning new things		
I can navigate my learning without somebody telling me what to do		
I am naturally curious		
I am open-minded		
I have a positive attitude about learning		
I ask "how" and "why" to work things out before I google		
When I disagree with someone, I try to understand their perspective		
When something doesn't go right, I ask "why" and try to learn from my mistakes		
I would rather "earn" a B than cheat to get an a		
I think about my thinking and learning		
My open-mindedness and reflection make me more caring		

are well-equipped to use critical thinking as your foundation for learning.

If you answered "No" to many of these questions:

You can be intentional about improving your abilities to be a critical thinker. Strengthening your critical thinking will support your academic success and prepare you for the complex decision making required in nursing practice.

Critical thinking is a foundation for your success in nursing school. Recognizing your areas for improving your critical thinking is a first step toward your success. ◄

1.3 Characteristics of Critical Thinkers

Understanding the characteristics of critical thinkers will help you integrate your critical thinking self-assessment into your attempts to improve your critical thinking. As we review these characteristics, we will look at examples of how a nursing student, Alba, applies these characteristics to her learning approach in nursing school.

- **Critical thinkers enjoy the process of learning**

Critical thinkers find joy in learning. This is particularly important to keep in mind as you journey through nursing school if you find yourself in a slump about your learning. A bad attitude interferes with your ability to learn and link new information to what you have previously learned. It is important not to let your attitude get in the way of being your best critical thinking self!

- **Critical thinkers are self-directed learners**

Critical thinkers embrace learning over performance. They actively engage in the work to learn and understand. A critical thinker will not be tempted to passively absorb information or shortcut learning for the sake of a good grade or getting an assignment off the "to do" list. Instead, a critical thinker will see each element of nursing school as a learning opportunity.

> **Example:**
>
> Nursing students are in a class being taught by an inexperienced and ineffective instructor. (It happens right? Every instructor can't be great.) Students complain and rally classmates to skip class saying things like "We don't learn anything anyway, why go?" Alba does not engage with this conversation. As a critical thinking student, Alba recognizes that class time, even with a less than stellar instructor, offers the opportunity to integrate previously learned concepts. She commits to spending extra time outside of class using active learning strategies to make meaningful connections with the course content. She will continue to resist joining in criticizing the instructor and instead put energy into learning with a mindset such as "I will have to work harder in this course because I'm not getting what I need from the instructor but in the long run the challenge will help me to be more self-sufficient in my learning." ◄

1.3 Characteristics of Critical Thinkers

- **Critical thinkers are curious**

Critical thinkers are eager to commit to deep learning; connecting new information to previously learned information with an eagerness to apply learning to new situations. A critical thinker who doesn't understand something will dig and probe further to assure their understanding. They approach every situation with a spirit of inquiry.

Example:

In a lecture about Coronary Artery Bypass Grafting (CABG), Abla struggles to understand how CABG improves circulation to the heart muscle. Instead of ignoring the issue in hopes of it not being relevant for an exam, she takes initiative. She recognizes this as a knowledge gap and actively addresses it. First she revisits their course readings and reviews the anatomy of the heart. She knows she learns best with visual representations so she searches for a video that includes a diagram and detailed explanation of CABG. After putting it all together in her mind, she draws a concept map. Now Alba has a comprehensive understanding of the topic and can answer the question "how does CABG improve circulation to the heart muscle?" This deeper understanding will help the student answer other questions about CABG and nursing care as it relates to the procedure. ◄

(Don't panic if you don't understand what CABG is as you read this; you will learn it in one of your future nursing courses. The important point here is that the student used critical thinking to learn and understand instead of just focusing on "will this be on the exam.")

- **Critical thinkers are open-minded**

Critical thinkers are willing to consider new ways of doing things, and willing to consider alternate attitudes about and approaches to situations. A critical thinker cannot accept "we've always done it that way" as a reason for doing something, recognizing that not every situation adheres to the same set of rules. They are open to considering new strategies and innovations.

Being open-minded requires commitment to this way of thinking. If you grew up in an environment that did not embrace open-mindedness, you may have to be more intentional about shifting your thinking to embracing new and even sometimes opposing ideas.

Example:

Alba is learning about wound care techniques in the first nursing clinical course. The instructor has taught aseptic and sterile dressing change techniques, and the students are required to perform a return demonstration of each in the skills lab. In clinical the next day, Alba observes a nurse in the unit using a slightly different approach for an aseptic dressing change. Instead of criticizing this nurse for not following procedure, Alba is open-minded and willing to consider there may be something she doesn't understand about why the nurse would deviate from what Alba did in the skills lab. As she thinks it through, she realizes the nurse did maintain asepsis but had to modify it because of the supplies that were available. Alba recognized that different situations may require varied wound care techniques. ◄

- **Critical thinkers have a positive attitude about learning**

Critical thinkers consider learning as an opportunity and not a chore and understand that attitude influences learning. They embrace pieces of new information as building blocks that expand the mind, allowing for synthesis of new information with what is already learned while maintaining a positive attitude about the opportunity to learn.

Example:

Students are assigned a simulation focusing on therapeutic communication with a client admitted for end of life care. Alba is assigned to the first group of students who must prepare for and complete the simulation before the class lecture on end-of-life care. While many students might complain about this scheduling issue, Alba sees this as an opportunity rather than a setback. Recognizing the value of a positive attitude in enhancing learning, she embraces the challenge and begins by reviewing prior related learning. She reviews class notes and readings from the class on therapeutic communication and course readings on end-of-life care. Alba prepares for the simulation by thinking about how the principles of therapeutic communication in nursing apply in end-of-life care. She reflects on her recent life experience; her grandmother who she loved dearly passed away last year while in the hospital. Alba reflects on how her family felt during that time and what their needs were. Even though this reflection elicits sad feelings, she can remain positive as she considers how this experience can apply to her learning. She synthesizes all of this learning to prepare for the simulation. ◄

- **Critical thinkers answer the "why" and "how"**

Critical thinkers consistently ask "why" and "how" to enhance their understanding. They do not settle for surface-level explanations but strive to achieve a deep understanding of the topic. This approach leads not just to a better understanding of content, but also supports the ability to apply learning to similar and related situations.

Example:

Alba is studying content on Type 1 and Type 2 Diabetes. In her class notes she has written "Type 1—always on insulin" and "Type 2—start with lifestyle change, then meds, insulin later."

Alba is reviewing her notes after class and realizes she does not understand "why," if they are the same disease, Type 1 is managed differently than Type 2. Drawing on their prior

learning and personal experience, she delves deeper striving to understand. She had a classmate in high school who had diabetes and used an insulin pump. Her grandmother who recently passed away also had diabetes but did not start insulin until about a year before she passed. Alba knows she needs to distinguish these two types of diabetes from a physiological level.

She goes back through course readings and engages in critical analysis of the information. In Type 1 diabetes, the pancreas fails to produce insulin. In Type 2, the pancreas may be producing less insulin but the issue is insulin resistance in the body's cells. This explains why a client with Type 1 diabetes would be on insulin and use a pump for consistent low doses of insulin, whereas a client with Type 2 diabetes can make changes in diet and lifestyle and use medications before going on insulin. The difference in insulin resistance also explains why the person with Type 2 diabetes is on higher doses of insulin.

Now Alba can understand the difference well enough that she could even explain it to another nursing student. ◄

- **Critical thinkers prioritize learning over achievement**

Critical thinkers value the process of learning over achieving grades or getting assignments completed. They know understanding and achieving competency is important because nursing knowledge is cumulative, building from one course to the next.

Example:

Students are required to submit handwritten remediation for standardized tests (course and subject tests in the NCLEX prep product). This handwritten remediation is submitted to the course instructor to receive the exam grade. There are rumors from students who took the course previously that the instructor doesn't look at the remediation assignments, just checks they are done and enters the grade.

1.3 Characteristics of Critical Thinkers

Some students in the class handwrite word for word the question rationale to complete the assignment. They are not learning the content, they are simply writing the rationale to complete the assignment.

Using her critical thinking Alba recognizes this approach of writing rationale without understanding the content will not support her learning. She also understands this approach will interfere with her ability to apply what she can learn from remediation in other ways, like course exams, in clinical or simulation. She will make time to remediate in a way that assures learning and understanding. It will take more time but her desire to understand will override the temptation to take shortcuts. ◄

- **Critical thinkers reflect on their learning**

Reflection on learning enhances both critical thinking and long-term assimilation of learned information. This is why nursing students often have clinical assignments that include reflective journals, post-conferences at the end of a clinical day, and debriefing after simulation. Reflection on learning supports synthesis and integration of learning that enhances understanding.

Example:

Alba is in a group of students assigned with an in-class project of creating a concept map relating two related diseases; Cushing's syndrome and Addison's disease. When the concept maps were presented, Alba recognized that her groups' concept map was missing the most important key elements that characterized the interconnectedness of the diseases; one involving excessive production of adrenal hormones (Cushing's syndrome) and the other characterized by insufficient production (Addison's disease). Alba's group had listed signs and symptoms of each without relating them to adrenal function. Rather than brush it off as an embarrassing event, Alba will take

time after class for reflection to understand what went wrong and identifies contributing factors:

(a) Lack of preparation—she had only skimmed the endocrine disorders readings that were part of class preparation. The same was true for other members in her group, because like Alba, they focused last evening on preparing for an exam in another class instead of preparing for this class.
(b) Critical thinking skills—her lack of preparation was a stressor as she tried to work with the group. This reduced her ability to use thinking skills to link pieces of information together.
(c) Group dynamics—the group members were more focused on finishing their concept map quickly to allow time to study for the exam that was being given in their next class.

This reflection on learning helped Alba see that preparation for class was the major contributing factor. With further reflection she realized the other groups' concepts maps that linked the adrenal hormone enhancing understanding of the two diseases. ◄

- **Critical thinkers translate their learning into caring behavior**

Caring and compassion is the outcome of a genuine desire to understand all aspects of a client's condition. Critical thinkers recognize that a comprehensive understanding of the client and the client's condition improves their ability to provide empathetic and compassionate care. Dedication to critical thinking fosters a deeper understanding of nursing practice and improves the quality of care nurses provide.

Now that you have learned about the characteristics of critical thinking, complete the Pause and Reflect 1.2 My Critical Thinking Journey. Consider these in relation to your critical thinking Self-Assessment 1.1.

▶ **Pause and Reflect 1.2: My Critical Thinking Journey** Write your responses to the following questions.

1. Which characteristic of critical thinkers do you feel are your strongest?
2. Which do you think you need to develop further? Why?

Remember, your ability to think critically is not a fixed ability. Striving to adopt characteristics of critical thinking will help you improve in your learning and your ability to think like a nurse.

Nursing School Application: Critical Thinking in Simulation

Critical thinking is an important habit to adopt as you navigate through nursing school and prepare to become a nurse. Let's look at how Alba uses critical thinking in simulation.

Students in Alba's class are preparing for a simulation lab on the concept of oxygenation. They are given the following pre-reading instructions:

Simulation Overview:

For this simulation, you will assess a client for oxygenation status and initiate appropriate intervention.

Client Profile:

- Client Name: Mr. John Smith
- Age: 72 years
- Gender: Male
- Past Medical History: Arteriosclerotic Cardiovascular Disease (ASCVD), Chronic Obstructive Pulmonary Disease (COPD), and Benign Prostatic Hypertrophy (BPH)
- Reason for admission: Pneumonia

Simulation Steps:

1. **Initial Assessment:**
   - Upon entering the room, observe the client's overall appearance, skin color, and respiratory rate.
   - Note any signs of distress, use of accessory muscles, or audible wheezing.
2. **Vital Signs:**
   - Measure vital signs
     - Vital signs will be provided as assessment is conducted.
3. **Physical Examination:**
   - Perform a thorough respiratory assessment, including:
     - Inspection: Observe the chest for any retractions, deformities, or unequal expansion.
     - Palpation: Assess for tactile fremitus and chest expansion.
     - Percussion: Evaluate for hyper-resonance or dullness.
     - Auscultation: Listen to lung sounds using a stethoscope and identify any wheezing, crackles, or diminished breath sounds.
4. **Oxygen Administration Decision:**
   - Based on assessment findings determine if the client requires supplemental oxygen and if oxygen is indicated, determine the appropriate delivery method and flow rate.
5. **Intervention:**
   - If oxygen is to be delivered, set up the oxygen delivery system and adjust the flow rate.
   - Ensure proper positioning and comfort for the client while administering oxygen.
6. **Evaluation:**
   - Stay in the room and maintain therapeutic communication as you assess the client's response to your intervention.
   - Monitor vital signs, SpO2, and respiratory effort.
   - Determine if change in the treatment plan is indicated and if so, initiate change.
   - Document findings, interventions, and evaluation of intervention.
7. **Client Education:**
   - Educate Mr. Smith about treatment.

When preparing for the simulation Abla does the preparation understanding that she will need to consider each of the diagnoses and what each means for oxygenation. She is focused on answering the "why."

Alba remembers the lecture on oxygen and COPD and writes a note that you can't give high oxygen to clients with COPD. She looked that up after class because she didn't understand why that would be. Because she took time to learn it well enough to explain the "why" she is able to remember now both the reason (with COPD, respiratory drive is based on low levels or oxygen because the body adjusts to the lower levels. When oxygen levels drop, a client with COPD will be at risk because when oxygen levels go up, they will breathe less. This is the opposite of normal.) and the intervention (give only 1–2 Liters if needed and if more respiratory support is needed the client will have to have positive pressure ventilation). She doesn't even need to review her notes; because she learned and understood the "why" she was able to recall it for the simulation. She is prepared to pay attention to oxygen delivery based on his COPD diagnosis when she does the simulation tomorrow.

In the simulation, Alba has confidence but also knows this is a learning experience. She is prepared and composed when she enters the room and begins her nursing assessment and care. She is not alarmed by his pulse ox of 88% with the diagnosis of COPD. She continues her respiratory assessment and reassures the client while she completes the assessment. She starts oxygen at 1 L via nasal cannula, elevates the head of the bed to 45 degrees, and converses with the client while she continues to monitor respiratory status.

In the simulation debriefing, Alba reflects on her performance and learning. She shared how in her prep, she reviewed COPD diagnosis and recognized it as important related to oxygenation. When she evaluated her learning, she reflected that she did the correct nursing intervention but did not remember to assess Mr. Smith's understanding of the situation and his care.

She applied critical thinking to her preparation, during the simulation and in the debriefing.

You may relate to Alba's approach to the simulation; perhaps your self-assessment revealed to you that you already have good critical thinking skills you are applying in nursing school. If, however, you don't have a solid critical thinking approach, there are practical strategies you can use to develop your skills.

1.4 Practical Strategies for Critical Thinking

Critical thinking is not a natural-born talent. It is a skill that anyone can learn and improve with practice. Even if you don't currently identify with the characteristics of a critical thinker, you can develop these traits by adopting specific strategies.

- **Think about thinking**

Critical thinking is just that, thinking. Reflect on your learning, think about what you are learning, think about connecting content to what you already know. When something that is not clear to you, gather more information and think about it. Try to generate your own "why" and "how" questions and work out the answers yourself. The more you do this, the more it will become your way of thinking.

- **Prioritize learning over performance**

A critical thinking mindset will enhance your learning while also improving your performance. It is a challenge in nursing school when you have multiple priorities for assignments and deadlines.

It is important to put thinking first; to prioritize thinking and understanding over completing tasks.

- **Discover your best way of learning and lean into it**

You may already know how you learn best. Learning can be primarily visual (reading), auditory (hearing), kinesthetic (moving), or psychomotor (doing). You can find online sources for assessing your learning style, but you probably already have figured out the conditions under which you learn best.

Leverage your learning style to help apply critical thinking in your learning. If your learning style is auditory, listen to recordings of your lecture after class. If kinesthetic, listen to recordings of lectures while you are taking a walk. If you are visual, look for images and videos that will supplement your learning in class.

- **Manage your time**

When you cut yourself short on time you will be inclined to go into survival mode and not make time for your learning. Use critical thinking to determine how you can be more productive with your time. Practicing critical thinking requires time to reflect on learning, explore new information on your own, and sit with your learning as you process and develop understanding of what you are learning.

- **Curate an open mind**

Conduct a self-assessment of biases and judgments that influence how you receive and learn information. Recognize that your life experience has shaped these biases and for the most part, they are implicit, meaning, you aren't aware that they exist and are shaping your attitudes and learning. You can begin by assessing your biases about race and gender by completing this *Implicit Bias Test* and review your results

- **Seek diverse perspectives**

Embrace alternative views and ideas as part of your critical thinking. Instead of dismissing something new, commit to learning more about it and draw conclusions about the validity of new things based on your critical thinking and not on judgments.

- **Stay positive about learning**

Because learning has two dimensions; cognitive and affective, your critical thinking is rooted in your attitudes about learning. Critical thinking improves when positive thoughts are linked to the learning experiences. Keep your attitude in check. A better attitude equals better thinking and learning.

- **Reflect on learning**

Reflection while you are learning, and after a learning experience, are essential for critical thinking. Reflect on what you are learning while you study, attend class, or go to clinical. Reflect on how you link new learning to previously learned information. Reflect on learning that comes easily (most likely will be topics that you enjoy) and reflect on your challenges. If you did not do well on an exam, reflect on "why" and identify areas for improvement. Consider alternate approaches and when you try them, reflect on how well they worked.

- **Ask "what if"**

Application of content you are learning is applied to various situations. This is an important aspect of a nurse's clinical judgment. In nursing school, you will apply information you learn to other scenarios; on exam questions, in your simulation and clinical experiences. Critical thinking helps you to adjust and apply what you know to similar and related situations.

- **Cluster-related information**

When you learn new information, identify other pieces of information that are related, and identify how they relate. Is one of these things not like the other? What things are similar, what things are different? Asking these questions will develop your critical thinking.

- **Ask "why" and "how"**

Create a habit of asking probing questions to deepen your understanding of concepts and experiences. Instead of accepting information at face value, uncover underlying reasons. Use active learning to explore these answers for yourself.

1.5 Critical Thinking Links to Clinical Decision Making and Clinical Judgment

Let's go back to where we started, looking at the Tanner's Model (Fig. 1.2) that depicts thinking in nursing. How will your critical thinking "habits" support your development of clinical decision making and clinical judgment?

1.5.1 Noticing

When you are noticing, you are considering all the "cues" you need to understand what might be happening with the client. You will think about this process and understand that in this first step, you need to attend to information from various sources and think about how that information fits together and is related.

You link what you know about the client's diagnosis and medical history to your previous learning and think about that as you complete your collection of client data. Think about what you are noticing (in the client chart and by looking at the clients) and think about what else you need to notice.

Think about biases that influence your observations. Listen (or read, if it is an unfolding care study or simulation pre-read) carefully and stay open-minded to notice everything that is important.

1.5.2 Interpreting

Because critical thinking is your habit, you will be able to analyze important "cues" and apply that to everything you have learned as it relates to this client. You will use your thinking to analyze the data and determine what it means in relation to the client's clinical condition.

What is the setting? Is the client stable? Are there urgent unmet needs that require immediate intervention? What will be the priority intervention? Are there other diagnoses that will change the expected findings for the main diagnosis?

You are using your critical thinking to link your learning about the presenting disease or condition, the circumstances of the setting, and your hypothesis about the care needs. You will reflect on your learning in the process. Is there an important "cue" that is missing? Have you gathered all the information needed in order to make the most accurate interpretation of the data?

1.5.3 Responding

Your critical thinking has provided a basis for your clinical decision making and now you will carry out your nursing intervention (clinical judgment). Because you have been intentional about your thinking throughout the process, you are able to respond using sound clinical decision making.

As you respond, you continue to reflect; is the initial client response what was expected? What is the appropriate amount of time to expect a change based on the initial response? Does the plan for intervention need to be altered based on that client response.

1.5.4 Reflecting

Reflecting is your thinking while you are in the process (reflecting in action) and after you complete the clinical interaction (reflecting on action). You are continually thinking throughout the process asking yourself the following questions. Table 1.3 Reflection Questions provides you with examples for questions that can lead your reflection in action and your reflection on action.

Linking critical thinking to Tanner's Model will help you as you move through your learning in nursing school.

Table 1.3 Reflection questions

Reflection IN action questions	Reflection ON action questions
Am I noticing any unexpected changes?	Did my initial assessment capture all relevant information?
What do the "cues" indicate?	How did my decisions and actions during the clinical interaction align with evidence-based practice guidelines?
Are there potential safety risks I need to address immediately?	Were there any missed opportunities for collaboration?
What additional information do I need?	Did I effectively prioritize and manage client care needs?
How effectively am I communicating with the client, family, and care team?	What aspects of my communication could have been improved?
Am I managing my emotions and stress?	Did my personal beliefs or values impact my performance?
What assumptions or biases might be influencing my perception of the situation?	What learning opportunities emerged from this experience?
How can I adapt my approach or interventions based on real-time feedback from my instructor?	How can I apply what I learned to future practice?

1.6   Conclusion

In this chapter, you've learned that critical thinking is the basic building block for nursing practice. Critical thinking takes you beyond memorizing facts to help you learn to think like a nurse; analyzing situations, making clinical decisions, and carrying out care. You can improve your critical thinking skills by embracing the characteristics of critical thinkers. Strengthening your critical thinking skills will support your success in nursing school in every aspect of your nursing school journey and into your nursing practice.

In the next chapter, we will delve into how the brain processes information and how this understanding can further support and enhance your critical thinking. Understanding the brain's role ("how" and "why") in learning will help you to commit to learning habits that lead to brain-based learning and success.

Chapter 1 Synthesis Learning Activity: Test Your "How" and "Why" Critical Thinking
This activity is designed to help you apply critical thinking as discussed in this chapter. Think back to your most recent experience in clinical, simulation, or skills lab. Write down the actions you took for each step in Tanner's Model related to the care your provided:

Noticing
Interpreting
Responding
Reflecting

Critical Thinkers strive to understand "how" and "why" and this understanding deepens their learning. Answer these questions using critical thinking. Consider the question and generate hypotheses before you look at the answers on the next page.

1. The client who has had a liver biopsy will be positioned on the right side. Why does this positioning prevent complications from the liver biopsy?
2. Wheezing is a continuous high pitched musical sound that is expiratory. Why is wheezing heard on expiration and not on inspiration?
3. How does a pulse oximeter measure oxygen levels in the blood?
4. A surgical incision heals from deep tissue layers to the skin surface. Why is this pattern of healing essential for preventing complications?

Answers to Test Your Critical Thinking questions. Were you able to apply your previous learning to generate hypotheses before you looked at the answer?

1. Placing the client on the right side helps to apply pressure to the biopsy site on the liver. This pressure assists in achieving hemostasis by promoting the formation of a blood clot at the puncture site, thereby reducing the risk of bleeding.
2. Wheezing occurs when the lower airways (bronchioles) are inflamed. This inflammation reduces the size of the airways. On exhalation, air is being pushed out of the lungs through the narrowed airways, which causes turbulence. On inhalation, air coming in is more passive and so there is less resistance.
3. A pulse oximeter measures oxygen levels by using light to detect how much oxygen is attached to the red blood cells as they pass through a small blood vessel, usually in the finger.
4. This pattern of healing is necessary because it prevents spaces or pockets from forming under the skin where fluid could collect and bacteria could grow. The body forms granulation tissue starting in the deepest layer of the wound, gradually building up layer by layer while maintaining blood supply throughout.

References

Caputi, L. (2017a). The why behind the what. *Nurse Educator, 42*(4), 163–163. https://doi.org/10.1097/NNE.0000000000000373

Caputi, L. J., & Kavanagh, J. M. (2018). Want your graduates to succeed? Teach them to think! *Nursing Education Perspectives, 39*(1), 2–3. https://doi.org/10.1097/01.NEP.0000000000000271

Dickison, P., Haerling, K. A., & Lasater, K. (2019). Integrating the National Council of State Boards of Nursing Clinical Judgment Model into nursing educational frameworks. *Journal of Nursing Education, 58*(2), 72–78. https://doi-org.ezproxy.ycp.edu:8443/10.3928/01484834-20190122-03

Lasater, K. (2007). Clinical judgment development: Using simulation to create an assessment rubric. *Journal of Nursing Education, 46*(11), 496–503. https://doi-org.ezproxy.ycp.edu:8443/10.3928/01484834-20071101-04

Scheffer, B. K., & Rubenfeld, M. G. (2000). A consensus statement on critical thinking in nursing. *The Journal of Nursing Education, 39*(8), 352–359. https://doi.org/10.3928/0148-4834-20001101-06

Tanner, C. A. (2006). Thinking like a nurse: A research-based model of clinical judgment in nursing. *Journal of Nursing Education, 45*(6), 204–211. https://doi.org/10.3928/01484834-20060601-04

Further Reading

Berg, C., Philipp, R., & Taff, S. D. (2023). Scoping review of critical thinking literature in healthcare education. *Occupational Therapy in Health Care, 37*(1), 18–39. https://doi.org/10.1080/07380577.2021.1879411

Caputi, L. (2017b). Guest editorial. The why behind the what. *Nurse Educator, 42*(4), 163. https://doi.org/10.1097/NNE.0000000000000373

Hans, J. (2024). Improving self-awareness and critical thinking through reflective practice. *British Journal of Community Nursing, 29*, S43–S46. https://doi.org/10.12968/bjcn.2024.0096

İlaslan, E., Adıbelli, D., Teskereci, G., & Üzen Cura, Ş. (2023). Development of nursing students' critical thinking and clinical decision-making skills. *Teaching & Learning in Nursing, 18*(1), 152–159. https://doi.org/10.1016/j.teln.2022.07.004

Patricia, K. M., Kabwe, C., Wamunyima, M. M., Margaret, M. M., & Dianna, J. L. (2022). Evidence based practice and critical thinking in nursing education and practice: A scoping review of literature. *International Journal of Nursing and Midwifery, 14*(4), 65–80. https://doi.org/10.5897/IJNM2022.0511

Ward, T. D., & Morris, T. (2016). Think like a nurse: A critical thinking initiative. *ABNF Journal, 27*(3). PMID 29443469.

Brain-Based Learning: Support Critical Thinking with Brain-Based Learning Strategies

2

Tell me and I will forget, show me and I may remember; involve me and I will understand.
—Confucius

2.1 Introduction

When you understand how your brain processes learning and why certain aspects of your behavior impact that learning, you can apply critical thinking to make changes that will improve your ability to learn and apply knowledge. This chapter introduces you to brain-based learning that involves learning with the natural functioning of your brain. By grasping these principles, you'll be better equipped to absorb, retain, and apply the vast amount of knowledge required in nursing school and throughout your career. We'll explore how critical thinking integrates with brain-based learning, and why your nursing program emphasizes teaching methods that support this approach.

▶ **By the end of this chapter you will be able to:**
1. Define brain-based learning and its relevance to nursing education.
2. Explain the connection between critical thinking and brain-based learning.
3. Understand neurophysiology related to effective learning and memory formation.
4. Identify brain-based learning strategies used in nursing education.
5. Apply brain-based learning techniques to enhance your study practices and information retention.

2.2 Brain-Based Learning

Critical thinking is integral to brain-based learning. It enables us to apply what we read, learn, and experience by connecting new information to what we have previously learned and transfer it to long-term memory. The other important aspect of brain-based learning for nursing school success is retrieval and application of learned information. You use your critical thinking and apply your learning when you take quizzes and exams, in simulation, in clinical, on NCLEX, and in nursing practice. This is why your nursing program is delivering content in a way that supports your brain-based learning.

Brain-based learning has been embraced by nursing education (Cardoza, 2011) because evidence suggests traditional methods of lecture and testing do not teach students to think like a nurse (Kavanagh, 2021). Your nursing instructors have probably attended workshops and are applying

---

© The Author(s), under exclusive license to Springer Nature Switzerland AG 2025
C. Thompson, *Nursing School, NCLEX and Career Transition Success*,
https://doi.org/10.1007/978-3-031-85538-2_2

teaching strategies that support brain-based learning in your classes and include:

- Flipped classroom
- Case studies
- Hands on learning activities during class
- Concept maps
- Simulation
- Problem solving activities

These teaching strategies can be frustrating if you prefer to listen to a lecture, take notes and memorize content for an exam. This process may help you feel more confident about an exam, but it does not support brain-based learning.

2.2.1 The Neurophysiology of Brain-Based Learning

Brain-based learning aligns learning with neurophysiology of the brain; how the brain naturally processes, stores, integrates, and recalls information.

Committing to learning strategies that support brain-based learning will be easier for you when you understand this neurophysiology.

Brain-based learning goes beyond memorization. While yes, there is some content you just must memorize in nursing school, brain-based learning enhances your ability to think like a nurse.

The building blocks for learning are neurons. You learned about them in Anatomy & Physiology. Let's briefly review them here.

Neurons are responsible for transmitting information throughout the brain and body. Each neuron consists of dendrites that receive information, axons that transmit signals, and cell bodies that house the neuron's core functions (Figs. 2.1 and 2.2).

Neurons communicate with one another across the synapse. Chemical messengers known as neurotransmitters play a pivotal role in transmission signals (bits of information) across the synapse. The neurotransmitters carry information through the brain, sorting and organizing it with related information, moving it to different parts of the brain and securing information into long-term memory.

Different neurotransmitters influence various aspects of learning and memory. For instance, serotonin is a neurotransmitter associated with

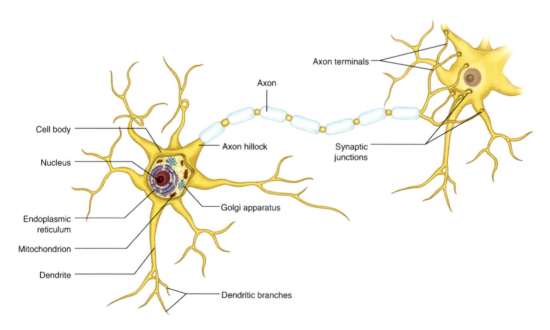

Fig. 2.1 Diagram of a neuron. (With permission from: George and Demesmin (2019))

2.2 Brain-Based Learning

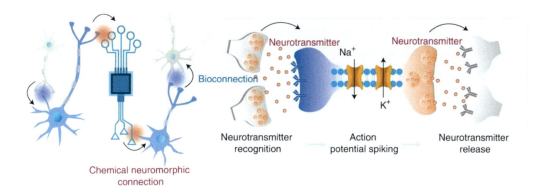

Fig. 2.2 Neuron to neuron synapse communication. (With permission from: Wang et al. (2022))

mood and emotional learning, while acetylcholine is crucial for memory formation.

Different parts of the brain work together in processing and storing information. The prefrontal cortex handles advanced thinking, like critical thinking. The hippocampus deals with memory processing. The amygdala connects emotions to learning (more on that later) and the basal ganglia aids in skill learning.

Learning occurs as the brain senses new information, integrates it into known data, moves it into short- and long-term memory (retention) and retrieves it to apply to repeated, related, or new experiences (Jensen & McConchie, 2020).

2.2.2 Brain-Based Learning Concepts

Your instructors are most likely using teaching strategies that support brain-based learning. These strategies include interleaving, repetition, chunking, and reflection (Churches et al., 2017). Let's review some of the aspects of brain-based learning.

- **Interleaving** is an aspect of brain-based learning that relies on scaffolding of information. You begin with introductory components of a concept and as you add higher level application, neurotransmitters link learned bits of information together. Your nursing school curriculum is based on this aspect of brain-based learning. You begin with introductory concepts and build on those throughout your coursework. This is a compelling reason to stay engaged in your learning, so that you can effectively link what is being taught in higher level courses to the learning from lower level courses.
- **Repetition** enhances brain-based learning as neurotransmitters reinforce movement and storage of information. This is why reading before class is vital to brain-based learning; you are repeating it with new and related information when the instructor reviews it in class, or when you apply it in a flipped classroom activity. This is also why reviewing your notes right after class, and repeatedly between the time it is presented and the time of the exam will support learning.
- **Chunking** enhances brain-based learning as neurotransmitters process information more effectively when information is reviewed in short bursts of activity, rather than in long periods of time. Dopamine and norepinephrine are released and activate neurotransmitters when learning segments are short, manageable, and engaging. The best way to "chunk" information is to stay focused on the learning for a short period of time. Evidence suggests 20 min per "chunk" is optimum before taking a break then continuing to another "chunk" of learning.
- **Reflection** stimulates neurotransmitters that reinforce learning and prioritizes learning. For example, when you care for a client your brain processes information that you learned during the experience. When you are reflecting on

your learning while you are in a learning situation, such as a simulation, and then reflect on your performance and learning after the simulation, you are boosting your learning and helping your brain to process learned material into long-term memory. You can apply this by thinking about your learning and stay actively engaged during clinical post-conference and simulation debriefing to reflect on your learning and on your performance.

The interaction of neurotransmitters throughout different *parts of the brain* controls learning and memory and plays a crucial role in thinking.

One part of the brain, the amygdala, connects emotions to learning, which explains how **attitude** impacts learning. This is why you remember more when you like the class or instructor. Even if you are in a course that is not your favorite, being mindful of the connection between attitude and learning will help you to stay calm, release serotonin, and enhance neurotransmitter activity. A positive attitude will help you learn AND remember what you are learning. Another way to improve your attitude about learning is to actively engage in your learning. Sitting in the front of the class, completing assignments without cutting corners, and staying positive about your ability to learn are all examples of ways to improve your attitude and enhance your learning (Jensen & McConchie, 2020).

Another part of your brain, the basal ganglia, aids in **skill learning**. This is why practicing a skill and putting the skill in a context of application helps you remember and perform better than reading a step by step list of how to perform the skill. This is also why skills lab, simulation, and clinical are valuable parts of your nursing school experience (Doyon & Benali, 2005).

Memory is a multifaceted phenomenon. Short-term memory is stored in the hippocampus. When you **sleep**, neurotransmitters move these memories from the hippocampus to the cortex of the brain. This function allows us to temporarily hold and manipulate information, while long-term memory is responsible for storing vast amounts of knowledge over extended periods. This highlights the importance of sleep as instrumental to enhancing brain-based learning (Rasch & Born, 2013).

Now that you understand how neurons, neurotransmitters, and different regions of the brain work together to process and store information, and how strategies like interleaving, repetition, chunking, and reflection enhance learning, take time to consider your own learning experiences. Consider handwriting your responses in a learning journal.

Complete Pause and Reflect 2.1 to examine how these brain-based learning principles may have already been working successfully for you, perhaps without you even realizing it.

> **Pause and Reflect 2.1: My Brain-Based Learning**
>
> Because you have learned the role of handwriting and reflection on enhancing your brain-based learning, you see the importance of the "'Pause and Reflect" journaling activities that are included throughout the book.
>
> For this Pause and Reflect, think about a recent learning experience where you felt you really understood and retained the information. Reflect on each question and write your reflections in a journal.
>
> 1. How did this experience align with the brain-based learning principles discussed?
> 2. Were elements of interleaving, repetition, or chunking involved?
> 3. How might you apply these principles to your future learning?
>
> When you understand the role of these actions on your learning, you can commit to applying them as you move through nursing school.

Nursing School Application: From Memorizing to Understanding: Brain-Based Approach to Learning BP Assessment

The instructor is introducing the topic of blood pressure (BP) assessment in the basic nursing course. We will look at how Alba, who applied critical thinking to her learning in Chap. 1, uses brain-based learning approaches with this topic.

The instructor included in the lecture the content in Table 2.1 BP Ranges and tells the students they need to know this content. Alba will make a note in class that she needs to know this and will create handwritten study notes on it after class.

The instructor reviewed causes of increased and decreased blood pressure and included Table 2.2 BP Comparison as part of the lecture notes.

Preparing for the skills lab, which takes place on the day following this class, the instructor reviews the procedure for proper BP assessment that is written in the lecture handout as a checklist:

BP Assessment Skills Checklist:

- Patient sitting
- Feet flat on floor
- Correct cuff size
- Center of cuff over brachial artery
- Lower end of cuff 1″ above antecubital space
- Cuff even and snug
- Inflate cuff
- Stethoscope over brachial artery in antecubital space
- Deflate cuff and listen for Korotkoff sounds

The instructor has provided handouts of the PowerPoint that includes these Tables and the checklist. Students who review the handout will move this content into their short-term memory, where it will remain for less than 24 h.

Alba will spend time after class reviewing the PowerPoint and the notes she took in class. Then she will apply her critical thinking for a better understanding and hand write her study notes. This enhances her brain-based learning, connecting the information to existing knowledge and promoting long-term retention.

The next day in the skills lab, students will practice BP assessment. This repetition and application to the learning in class the previous day will support transfer of the knowledge from short-term memory to long-term memory. Alba however will be further along because she has already linked her learning to her previous knowledge about the circulatory system. She does this by asking "why" questions and thinking through the answers. Below is her list of questions.

- WHY do heart problems cause high blood pressure?
- WHY does atherosclerosis cause high blood pressure?
- WHY do genetic factors cause high blood pressure?
- WHY does stress cause high blood pressure?
- WHY does smoking cause high blood pressure?

Alba's study notes, if they were written in a table, would include content outlined in Table 2.3 BP Critical Thinking.

Answering these questions gives Alba a deeper understanding of the content and allows her to retrieve learned information to apply it when she needs to think like a nurse answering exam questions, conducting simulation and in clinical.

You can apply Alba's brain-based learning in your nursing school journey. Take a few minutes to reflect on your strategies for brain-based learning and how you might improve as you complete Pause and Reflect 2.2; My Brain-Based Learning Action Plan.

Table 2.1 BP ranges

Category	Systolic		Diastolic
Normal	90–120	and	60–80
Low	<90	and	<60
Elevated	120–129	or	80–89
Stage 1 Hypertension	130–139	or	80–89
Stage 2 Hypertension	>140	or	>90
Hypertensive crisis	>180	or	>120

Table 2.2 BP comparison

Causes of high blood pressure	Causes of low blood pressure
Heart problems (e.g., coronary artery disease, heart valve disorders)	Heart problems (e.g., heart failure, bradycardia)
Atherosclerosis	Pregnancy
Genetics	Dehydration
Stress	Bed rest
Smoking	Blood loss

Table 2.3 BP critical thinking

Causes of high blood pressure	WHY
Heart problems	If the heart is having to push harder to get blood out, that harder push will result in a pressure against the arteries
Atherosclerosis	Atherosclerosis is "hardening of the arteries" from fats and changes to the wall of the artery. The thicker arteries are less resistant so blood pushing into them will have more resistance. It's like if you think about arteries as water balloons. If the balloon rubber is thicker, then the pressure has to be greater to get the blood to pass through the balloon
Genetic factors	Genes determine how blood pressure is regulated
Stress	Stress causes "fight or flight" meaning heart rate increases and blood vessels constrict. The arteries are more narrow so the pressure has to be greater for the blood to push through
Smoking	Chemicals in tobacco cause the heart rate to increase and blood vessels to constrict so same as stress

▶ **Pause and Reflect 2.2: My Brain-Based Learning Action Plan** Think about a challenging concept you've encountered in your nursing studies.

How could you apply brain-based learning strategies to better understand and remember this concept?

Create a brief study plan incorporating at least three of the strategies discussed in this chapter.

2.3 📝 Practical Strategies for Brain-Based Learning

Now that you understand how your brain processes and retains information, let's explore practical ways you can apply this knowledge to help you learn. These strategies work with your brain's natural learning processes, helping you absorb, retain, and recall information more effectively.

- **Maintain a positive attitude about learning**

When you approach your studies with enthusiasm and positivity, you improve your ability to remember.

Think back to something from your childhood that brings a smile to your face. Perhaps it was one of the happiest days of your childhood; a birthday party, a vacation, a time spent with someone special. Take a moment to reflect on this memory. Can you envision yourself right back in that moment? Can you see the entire scene in your mind? Can you hear the sounds, and can you recall the smells?

Most likely you can create a vivid multisensory picture of the experience because the experience was positive and happy.

Now, let's contrast this with a different day from your childhood, the one just before your happiest day. Can you remember anything specific about it? Chances are you can't. Why? There was no emo-

2.3 Practical Strategies for Brain-Based Learning

tional connection to that day, nothing to process and store the details into your long-term memory.

You can apply this to your nursing school journey by bringing enthusiasm into your learning and not allowing space for negativity or drudgery.

- **Embrace repetition**
  Your instructors will provide repeated content
  - Assigned reading before class
  - Content review in class; whether your class is lecture or flipped
  - Content reinforced in skills lab, simulation or clinical
  - Course exams
  - Standardized exams
  - Final exam

You will enhance your brain-based learning when you embrace the repetition of this content and understand that the content review supports your higher level learning. Even if you don't have an assignment like a quiz or "ticket to class" that requires you to do the pre-class readings, commit to doing them. Seeing the content a second time in class reinforces your learning. The more you review, the more you will learn.

- **Review class notes immediately after class**

Tempting as it is to leave class considering your work complete you will enhance your learning if you review key points from your class in a short burst of study time right after your class. Keep this in mind when you create your class schedule and when you plan other activities. Plan a short block of time to review your notes immediately after class.

- **Chunk your study time**

You likely already know that waiting until the day before an exam then "cramming" does not help you perform as well as when you keep up with the information over time. Even when you set aside study time, do your studying in chunks of time; most researchers recommend 20 min. Take a short break and then resume your studying.

- **Handwrite your notes**

Even though you've grown up using a computer and smartphone, and you may believe that typing notes during class works for you, our brains have not evolved to process typed information as efficiently as handwriting. Handwriting stimulates neurotransmitters that are not activated by typing. This is why handwriting reflections in a journal and handwriting your notes improves brain-based learning. The Cornell Method is an evidence-based note taking method that you may find helpful if you're not in the habit of using handwritten notes to enhance your learning.

- **Make sleep a priority**

The simple overview here is that you understand neurotransmitters work differently during your sleep cycles and in that work process what you have learned. It is an excellent way to boost your learning and enhance your long-term memory.

- **Add a psychomotor component to your learning**

This is the basis of some flipped classroom activities and of skills lab, simulation and clinical learning experience. Hands-on application experience enhances brain-based learning. When you understand the value of psychomotor learning activities you can embrace them with a learning attitude.

- **Avoid "task based" learning**

When you complete an assignment to "get it done" without paying attention to learning or understanding the content, you are not enhancing your brain's ability to process that information and make connections to relate it to other information and store it for later recall. Your goal is to apply learning to clinical scenarios. Strive to apply a context to the things you are learning.

• Don't cheat

We just have to say it and get it out there. Cheating does not in any way support brain-based learning. Across the spectrum of what cheating is, copying someone else's work, using AI to complete assignments, or getting answers to tests, cheating may help you get through a difficult moment, but it does not support brain-based learning.

• Reflect on your learning

You may have some assignments like clinical journals or simulation debriefing where you will be required to reflect on your learning, which support brain-based learning. Take it upon yourself to reflect on your learning even when it is not required; make reflection on learning an ongoing habit to support your brain-based learning. Table 2.4 Reflection Prompts provides examples

Table 2.4 Reflection prompts

CLASS
How actively did I participate in class?
What activities in class helped me understand the content?
What topics were difficult to grasp?
How can I create learning activities for myself to clarify the murky parts?
How well did my pre-class preparation help me understand the material?
What should I do after class to reinforce what I learned?
SIMULATION
How realistic did the simulation feel, and how did it enhance my learning?
How did I communicate and collaborate with my team during the simulation?
What connections did I make between classroom learning and simulation experience?
How did simulation help me apply theoretical knowledge to a practical situation?
CLINICAL
How confident did I feel during clinical today?
How could I have prepared for the activities I was not confident about today?
How well did I interact with my client and with my client's family?
How did I handle challenging situations?

of prompts to stimulate your reflective practices in your nursing school learning settings; class, simulation, and clinical.

You see there are a variety of strategies you can use to boost your brain-based learning; many that you likely are already using. By implementing these strategies, you can enhance your brain's ability to process, store, and retrieve information effectively, leading to improved performance in your nursing studies and future practice.

2.4 Conclusion

In this chapter, you've learned about the link between brain-based learning and critical thinking in nursing education. Understanding neurophysiology helps you adapt and commit to the learning strategies that your nursing instructors are asking you to use. Using these practical strategies such as embracing repetition, chunking study time, and reflecting on your learning, you can enhance your ability to absorb, retain knowledge. These strategies improve your ability to learn, remember what you learned, and apply your learning in nursing school, and just as importantly, in nursing practice.

The next chapter will review the concept of growth mindset and how it complements brain-based learning. You will discover how and why adopting a growth mindset allows you to become a more effective learner and how believing in your abilities improves your performance.

> **Chapter 2 Synthesis Learning Activity: Apply Brain-Based Learning**
> This activity is designed to help you apply the brain-based learning strategies discussed in this chapter to a specific nursing concept. By creating a personalized learning plan, you'll practice integrating these strategies into your study routine, enhancing your understanding and retention of important nursing knowledge.

(continued)

Choose a nursing concept you're currently studying or will study soon. Create a brain-based learning plan for this concept, incorporating at least five strategies discussed in this chapter. Your plan should include:

1. A brief description of the concept
2. How you will chunk the information
3. A strategy for interleaving this concept with previously learned material
4. A plan for repetition and review
5. A reflection component
6. A psychomotor or hands-on element (if applicable)

Explain how each part of your plan supports brain-based learning principles and how it will enhance your understanding and retention of the concept.

Churches, R., Dommett, E., & Devonshire, I. (2017). *Neuroscience for teachers: Applying research evidence from brain science*. Crown House Publishing Ltd..

Doyon, J., & Benali, H. (2005). Reorganization and plasticity in the adult brain during learning of motor skills. *Current Opinion in Neurobiology, 15*(2), 161–167. https://doi.org/10.1016/j.conb.2005.03.004

George, T., & Demesmin, D. (2019). Nerve function and neurons. In *Deer's treatment of pain*. Springer Nature. https://doi.org/10.1007/978-3-030-12281-2_4

Jensen, E., & McConchie, L. (2020). *Brain-based learning: Teaching the way students really learn*. Corwin Press.

Kavanagh, J. M. (2021). Crisis in competency: A defining moment in nursing education. *Online Journal of Issues in Nursing, 26*(1). https://doi.org/10.3912/OJIN.Vol26No01Man02

Rasch, B., & Born, J. (2013). About sleep's role in memory. *Physiological Reviews, 93*(2), 681–766. https://doi.org/10.1152/physrev.00032.2012

Wang, T., Wang, M., Wang, J., et al. (2022). A chemically mediated artificial neuron. *Nature Electronics, 5*, 586–595. https://doi.org/10.1038/s41928-022-00803-0

References

Cardoza, M. P. (2011). Neuroscience and simulation: An evolving theory of brain-based education. *Clinical Simulation in Nursing, 7*(6), e205–e208. https://doi.org/10.1016/j.ecns.2011.08.004

Neuroplasticity: Adopt a Growth Mindset to Power up Brain-Based Learning

3

It's not always the people who start out the smartest who end up the smartest.

—Carol S. Dweck, Mindset: How You Can Fulfill Your Potential

3.1 Introduction

Neuroplasticity is a game-changer for nursing students like you. It reveals that your brain's capacity for learning isn't fixed—it can grow and adapt with the right approach. Adopting a growth mindset and applying brain-based learning principles changes the very structure of your brain and improves your cognitive abilities. This is an exciting prospect for you as a nursing student, to learn how your thinking and approach to learning can actually make you smarter! This chapter will explore how embracing neuroplasticity and a growth mindset can help you navigate the challenges of nursing school more effectively, setting you up for success not just as a student, but as a lifelong learner and future nurse.

▶ **By the end of this chapter you will be able to:**
1. Define neuroplasticity and what it means for learning in nursing education.
2. Explain growth mindset and it relates to brain-based learning.
3. Understand how a growth mindset can improve cognitive abilities.
4. Identify challenges to maintaining a growth mindset in nursing school.
5. Apply growth mindset strategies throughout nursing education.
6. Recognize benefits of a growth mindset for nursing school and nursing career success.

When you understand how your brain can physically change in response to your experiences and learning, you can harness this power to become a more effective learner. This chapter introduces you to neuroplasticity and the growth mindset, two concepts that will revolutionize your approach to learning in nursing school and beyond.

3.2 Neuroplasticity: The Brain's Ability to Change

Neuroplasticity refers to the brain's remarkable ability to reorganize itself by forming new neural connections throughout life. This phenomenon allows the neurons (nerve cells) in the brain to compensate for injury and disease and to adjust their activities in response to new situations or changes in their environment (Kolb, 2013). Your brain is capable of physically changing its structure in response to learning and experience. This includes the growth of new neurons, a process

---

© The Author(s), under exclusive license to Springer Nature Switzerland AG 2025
C. Thompson, *Nursing School, NCLEX and Career Transition Success*,
https://doi.org/10.1007/978-3-031-85538-2_3

called neurogenesis, and the formation of new synaptic connections between neurons. These structural changes are accompanied by functional changes, where the brain can reassign roles to different regions. For instance, if one area is damaged, another may take over its functions (Gage, 2002).

We have long understood that at the synaptic level, the strength of connections between neurons can be increased or decreased based on how frequently they're used. The idea that "neurons that fire together, wire together" has been foundational to our understanding of synaptic plasticity. This concept, introduced by Hebb (2002) was originally published in 1949. Hebb's work laid the groundwork for our current understanding of how repeated activation strengthens neural pathways, emphasizing the role of repetition and practice in learning.

Your experiences, including learning new information or skills, directly influence these changes in your brain. This is known as experience-dependent plasticity. As you engage in your nursing studies, attend clinical rotations, and practice new skills, you're not just accumulating knowledge, you're physically reshaping your brain.

Neuroplasticity is relevant to you as a nursing student because it means your brain can continue to grow and adapt throughout your education and career (Lewis et al., 2024). It provides a biological basis for the idea that both your intelligence and abilities can be developed. This understanding is the "why" behind the importance of a growth mindset; when you believe your abilities can be developed through dedication and hard work, your brain changes to increase your capability for learning and understanding.

3.3 Growth Mindset

A growth mindset is the belief that your abilities, including your intelligence and talent, can be developed through effort, good strategies, and input from others (Dweck, 2006). This mindset aligns perfectly with the concept of neuroplasticity, as it encourages you to embrace challenges, persist in the face of setbacks, and view effort as the path to mastery. By cultivating a growth mindset, you're essentially promoting neuroplasticity in your brain, creating more neural connections and strengthening existing ones as you learn and grow.

However, maintaining a growth mindset throughout your nursing education isn't always easy. The demands and pressures of nursing school can challenge your belief in your ability to grow and improve. Let's explore why holding onto a growth mindset can be challenging in nursing school.

The rigor of nursing school can leave you feeling like a juggler juggling more balls in the air than you can handle. You need to focus on survival:

- **Daily survival**: A clinical day, a class presentation, an assignment due, a difficult exam.
- **Weekly survival**: A week filled with more than one exam or multiple big assignments like an exam and a presentation.
- **Semester survival**: In nursing school exam average can mean the difference between continuing or having to repeat a course. Worse yet, in most nursing schools, once you have not been successful in a second nursing course, you may be forced out of the program. Talk about pressure, right?

Beyond the demands of nursing school, you also have life. Gone are the days when students went off to nursing school with their only "job" being nursing school. You are most likely working, you have family responsibilities, and you have friends and other activities that keep you busy.

Being overwhelmed and busy pushes you against deadlines and leads you to complete assignments or prepare for exams just to get them done in time (performance) rather than to learn (growth). You lean into completing the most pressing and demanding work that is due, this day, this week, or this semester. In the pressure to get the work done you can overlook the learning that is key to supporting your growth mindset.

Before we explore strategies to develop and improve your growth mindset, let's take a moment for you to complete a Growth Mindset Self-Assessment.

Self-Assessment 3.1: Growth Mindset

The purpose of this self-assessment is for you to identify which attributes of a growth mindset you are already using. For each of the statements in Table 3.1 check Yes or No.

If you answered "Yes" to most of these questions:

You likely have a strong growth mindset, which is a valuable asset in your journey as a nursing student.

If you answered "No" to many of these questions:

You may have a more fixed mindset in certain areas, which can limit your potential for growth. Review the content in this chapter and apply your learning to cultivate a growth mindset.

Recognizing areas for growth is the first step toward developing a stronger growth mindset. Be honest with yourself, but also be kind. Every step toward a growth mindset is a step toward becoming a better learner (Williams, 2018, 2020).

Table 3.1 Growth mindset self-assessment

Growth mindset self-check	Yes	No
I see my mistakes as an opportunity to learn		
I believe my abilities can be developed through dedication and hard work		
I embrace challenges because they help me grow		
I persist in the face of setbacks		
I see effort as a path to mastery		
I learn from criticism and feedback		
I find inspiration in the success of others		
I believe intelligence can be developed over time		
I reflect on my learning process to improve		
I approach new tasks with a "can do" attitude		

Nursing School Application: Growth Versus Fixed Mindset
Students in their first semester of nursing courses are taking a Kaplan Practice Test in their Health Assessment class on a Friday. They are required to complete handwritten remediation for each question missed on the test. The hand written remediation is due the following Wednesday. Many students in the class have an exam in their other nursing course the following Monday, and clinical on Tuesday.

3.3.1 Fixed Mindset

Naomi's Nursing School Juggling Act
Naomi has a hectic schedule. She works two 12-hour shifts every other weekend to support herself while in school, and this particular weekend happens to be her work weekend. With her plate overflowing with responsibilities, Naomi faces a dilemma. She understands the importance of remediation for her learning, but time is limited so she makes a calculated decision. She is tired. She has had a long week and has to work the weekend. Her friends are getting together Friday evening and needing a break Naomi decides to take Friday afternoon and evening "off" from schoolwork.

After her work weekend, she prioritizes the Monday exam, clinical preparation, and Health Assessment class preparation over the Kaplan Practice Test remediation. Rushed for time Naomi completes the remediation assignment by glancing at the rationale for questions she answered incorrectly and rearranging wording for her handwritten remediation assignment.

Let's look at a question Naomi got incorrect and the fallout from that task oriented approach:

The nurse is assessing blood pressure and notes the BP in the right arm is 140/90 mm Hg, while the left arm reads 180/110 mm Hg.

(continued)

► **The nurse knows this may be indicative of which of the following?**
1. Deep vein thrombosis
2. Elevated blood glucose levels
3. Aortic dissection
4. Urinary tract infection

Naomi had selected (1) as the answer. She was able to rule out elevated blood glucose levels (2) and urinary tract infection (4), so she has to select between deep vein thrombosis (1) and aortic dissection (3).

She knew the aorta is in the circulatory system, but she never heard aortic dissection so she questioned if it was even a medical term. Because deep vein thrombosis is also a circulatory system and because she knew it was a real thing she selected it as the correct answer.

Now remediating the test and completing her assignment of handwriting remediation she reads the answer rationale:

> Differences in blood pressure readings between the arms could be caused by improper measure technique; differences in positioning of the arms, improper cuff placement or use of an improperly sized cuff. When proper measure technique is used, a significant difference in blood pressure readings between the arms, referred to as "arm-to-arm" blood pressure indicate a dissecting aorta, where the dissection disrupts blood flow to one of the arms, leading to varying blood pressure measurements. It is crucial for the nurse to recognize this difference and assess the client further for signs and symptoms of aortic dissection.

Naomi does not have time to look into this to understand it. She writes her remediation:

> A dissecting aorta can cause an "arm to arm" difference in blood pressure.

Now Naomi isn't able to explain "why" a dissecting aorta can lead to "arm to arm" differences and she will not have this in her long-term memory. In her rush to get her remediation assignment done she has missed out on a learning opportunity.

Fast forward. Naomi has finished nursing school, yeah! She has had bumps along the road, mostly because she was busy every semester with work and school and did more performing than learning.

Now Naomi is taking NCLEX and has this question on her exam:

A 60-year-old male client arrives at the emergency department with sudden, severe chest pain radiating to the back. On assessment, the nurse notes a significant difference in blood pressure between the right and left arms, with the right arm reading 140/90 mm Hg and the left arm reading 180/110 mm Hg.

► **Which assessment findings are related to a possible dissecting aortic aneurysm?**
1. Diminished breath sounds on the left side
2. Bruit over the abdominal aorta
3. A pulsatile mass in the abdomen
4. Bilateral pedal cyanosis
5. Tachycardia
6. Loss of consciousness

Naomi will miss this NCLEX question because she never learned this content well enough to understand it.

Fast Forward. Naomi is working in her first job in the Emergency Department. She has completed her orientation so she is on her own. She is assigned to care for the following client:

> Mr. X. is a 56-year-old male who presents to the Emergency Department (ED) with a complaint of chest pain. Naomi records Mr. X.'s vital signs and initiates the protocol for chest pain, performs the electrocardiogram (ECG), administers oxygen, nitroglycerin, and aspirin. She leaves the room to care for her other assigned clients. Because she did not address other cues that suggested Mr. X. had a dissecting aorta, by the time she returned to room 15 min later to reassess his chest pain, Mr. X. had lost consciousness and was in cardiac arrest. By the time his dissecting aorta was diagnosed he had lost so much blood that he did not survive surgery.

3.3.2 Growth Mindset

Alba Commits to Learning over Performance
Let's look again at Alba. You'll remember in Chap. 1 she demonstrated critical thinking. Just like Naomi, she has multiple demands on her time.

Alba knows that she will learn best if she does her remediation when the Kaplan Practice Test questions are fresh in her mind. She takes a break for lunch when she finishes the Practice Test and even though friends are getting together right after lunch, Alba goes to her quiet study space to complete her remediation.

When Alba reviews she is focusing on understanding it as it applies to how a nurse will use clinical judgment in nursing practice.

Alba knows she learns best with analogies. Like Naomi, she missed this question:

The nurse is assessing blood pressure and notes the BP in the right arm is 140/90 mm Hg, while the left arm reads 180/110 mm Hg.

▶ **The nurse knows this may be indicative of which of the following? (Select all that apply)**
1. Deep vein thrombosis
2. Elevated blood glucose levels
3. Aortic dissection
4. Urinary tract infection

Alba knows she needs to understand two topics—arm to arm difference and aortic dissection.

After learning the content, Alba writes this analogy to synthesize her learning.

The vascular system is like a highway that carries blood through the body. The heart beat propels blood evenly to both sides of the body. When there is a difference between the right and left side, something is wrong. The aorta is the body's main highway for blood coming out of the heart. If the inside lining of the aorta tears, blood goes into the tear and makes the force different. Because the inside lining is tearing the cli-

ent will have pain. More important than the arm to arm difference and pain is that this client could die. This is a MEDICAL EMERGENCY.

Now Alba has learned this content and because she understands it, she is more likely to remember it. When she gets an NCLEX question on this topic, she is able to apply her learning and answer it correctly. When she is the nurse in the ED and Mr. X. presents with chest pain. Alba will be able to provide safe and effective care as follows:

Alba, recognizing the urgency of chest pain, makes a clinical judgment to start oxygen and perform an electrocardiogram (ECG). Alba notes that Mr. X used the word "tearing" when he described his chest pain and realizes this is an important cue. She knows dissecting aorta can cause this. Because she adopted a growth mindset in her learning, Alba remembered dissecting aortic and is able to apply it to this clinical case. She understands dissecting aorta is a medical emergency. She quickly but thoroughly gathers more assessment data. Even though the chest pain protocol includes administration of nitroglycerin and aspirin, Alba is going to hold these medications and immediately notify the ED physician. A stat CT scan is ordered, the aneurysm is diagnosed and Mr. X. is transported for surgery.

Alba's commitment to a growth learning mindset in nursing school will save Mr. X's life.

Now you see the short-term and long-term implications of a growth mindset. It serves you in the immediate present time as you are learning and applying your learning while supporting your success in future nursing courses, on NCLEX and in your nursing practice. Take a moment to reflect on how you can activate your growth mindset by completing Pause and Reflect 3.1.

▶ Pause and Reflect 3.1: Activating My Growth Mindset

You may recall times you performed like Naomi, getting an assignment done on time without committing to a growth mindset to learn. Take a moment to reflect on the following:

1. Think about a time you approached a task or assignment with a fixed mindset, similar to Naomi. What was the outcome? How might the result have been different if you had adopted a growth mindset like Alba?
2. Identify one upcoming assignment or learning opportunity where you can apply a growth mindset. How will you approach it using a growth mindset instead of a fixed mindset?
3. Reflect on the connection between neuroplasticity, growth mindset, and lifelong learning in nursing. How does understanding this connection motivate you to approach your studies differently?

Every learning opportunity in nursing school contributes to your ability to provide safe and effective patient care. By adopting a growth mindset, you're not just improving your grades—you're laying the foundation for excellence in your nursing career.

3.4 📋 Practical Strategies: Create a Growth Mindset

Now that you understand the importance of a growth mindset, let's look at strategies to help you embrace a growth mindset, effectively "rewiring" your brain for improved learning and performance. Developing a growth mindset is a journey, not a destination. Be patient with yourself as you work to implement these strategies, and celebrate the progress you make along the way.

- **Identify your current mindset**

Earlier in this chapter, you completed a self-assessment and reflected on the results. Now that you have insight into whether you tend toward a growth or fixed mindset, it's time to take action.

If you already have a growth mindset, focus on reinforcing and strengthening it. If you lean more toward a fixed mindset, commit to adjusting your thinking patterns toward growth.

This step is crucial because your mindset profoundly impacts your ability to learn and succeed in nursing school. When you operate from a growth mindset, you actually get smarter! You improve your ability to:

- Learn new information effectively
- Apply your knowledge in various situations
- Develop robust critical thinking skills
- Perform better on tests and exams
- Prepare for your future nursing practice

Your mindset isn't set in stone. With conscious effort and practice, you can cultivate a growth mindset that will serve you well throughout your nursing education and career. By embracing this perspective, you're not just setting yourself up for success in school—you're laying the foundation for becoming a more adaptable, resilient, and effective nurse.

- **Embrace challenges**

Nursing school is challenging and sometimes you may feel like just giving up; you can't possibly understand what the instructor wants, or how to apply your learning on a test. Staying ahead of the challenge and facing it with an eagerness to overcome it and learn will support your growth mindset. Believe in your ability to address the challenges that each course brings your way. As you embrace your challenges, think about how great you will feel when you achieve your success!

- **Set incremental goals on your journey to success**

There's a saying, "How do you eat an elephant? One bite at a time." Nursing school can feel overwhelming especially in the beginning of the semester when you review everything that will be required in the semester. Instead of accepting the overall picture as a crushing weight, break it down into manageable tasks.

Writing a weekly calendar may help make getting through a semester less overwhelming. Each semester you complete, celebrate that you are one step closer to graduation.

- **Learn from feedback; both positive and negative**

Positive feedback is always fun and gives us an opportunity to feel good about our work and integrate our learning. On the other hand, it can be discouraging to get feedback that is negative; a test where you scored lower than you had hoped, a simulation where you missed an important cue about the client's condition, a clinical situation where you could have performed better. When you use a growth mindset, you see these as opportunities to learn and apply your learning to future situations.

- **Be persistent**

Dr. Seuss got 27 rejections on the first book he wrote for publication. His persistence in the face of repeated setbacks ultimately led to his becoming one of the most beloved children's authors of all time. This same spirit of perseverance is crucial in nursing school and will serve you well in your nursing career.

You will face challenges—difficult exams, complex clinical scenarios, and moments of self-doubt. These are not roadblocks, but stepping stones on your path to becoming a nurse. Each time you push through a difficult concept, overcome a challenging clinical day, or improve after a disappointing grade, you're building resilience and reinforcing your growth mindset.

- **Be inspired by others**

Finding inspiration in those around you can be a powerful motivator and support for your growth mindset. Look for role models and success stories in your nursing education journey and beyond:

(a) Faculty members: Do you have an instructor who has overcome challenges to become a great teacher? Perhaps they switched careers later in life, or overcame personal obstacles. Their journey can remind you that persistence pays off.

(b) Clinical nurses: Think about a nurse you observed during your clinical rotations who seemed to embody everything you aspire to be as a nurse. What qualities did they exhibit? How did they interact with patients and colleagues? Use their example as a goal to work toward.

(c) Classmates: Pay attention to your peers who are excelling or overcoming difficulties. Their strategies and attitudes might offer valuable lessons.

(d) Personal heroes: Is there someone in your life—a family member, friend, or public figure—whose accomplishments you admire? Their success in their field can inspire you in your nursing journey.

By drawing inspiration from others, you remind yourself of what's possible. Their stories can provide motivation during tough times and help you envision your own future success. One day you will be inspiring others!

- **Embrace the power of "not yet"**

When you encounter setbacks in your nursing education—whether it's not passing an exam, struggling to meet a competency in simulation or clinical, or even not passing a course—resist the urge to label these experiences as failures. Instead, adopt the powerful mindset of "not yet."

"Not yet" acknowledges that while you haven't achieved your goal at this moment, you're on a journey of growth and learning. It shifts your perspective from a fixed endpoint to a continuous process of development. This simple phrase can transform how you view challenges and setbacks, keeping you focused on improvement rather than getting stuck in self-doubt or disappointment. By embracing the power of "not yet," you're cultivating resilience, fostering a love of learning, and preparing yourself for the ongoing professional development that characterizes a successful nursing career.

- **Reflect on your performance to enhance your learning**

When you receive outcomes that are less than you hoped for, learn from those and apply that learning to your future endeavors. Use the prompts in Table 3.2 Performance Evaluation Feedback to guide your reframing negative feedback and challenges into opportunities for growth and learning.

There are a variety of strategies you can use to develop and maintain a growth mindset that begin with identifying your current mindset. By implementing more growth mindset strategies, you can cultivate your growth mindset and harness the power of neuroplasticity.

Table 3.2 Performance feedback reflection

Negative feedback	Growth mindset reflection
Not understanding an important concept	Have I sought out additional resources or explanations? Did I try to use critical thinking? Can I break this concept/skill down into smaller, more manageable parts? Am I practicing active recall and spaced repetition in my study of this topic?
Scoring poorly on an exam	Did I "chunk" my study time? Was this the first exam in the course; what can I learn about what the instructor emphasizes from the classes and notes? Did I manage my lifestyle strategies before the exam (get enough sleep, eat a healthy meal?) (Chap. 6) Did I manage my thoughts to maximize my focus and performance (Chap. 4)
Missed an important cue in simulation	Did I thoroughly prepare for the simulation? Was I focused on my thinking and recognizing cues in the assessment? What impacted my ability to recognize this cue?
Not meeting a competency in clinical	Was I adequately prepared for the clinical? Did I get sufficient sleep prior to the clinical? Was I distracted by something in the environment that contributed to my not recognizing best practice?

3.5 Conclusion

In this chapter, we've explored the concepts of neuroplasticity and growth mindset, understanding how they are connected and how they can enhance your learning potential. By adopting a growth mindset, you can actively promote neuroplasticity and create for yourself a positive cycle of learning and development. The challenges you face in nursing school are opportunities for growth, not indicators of fixed abilities (Jeffs et al., 2021). As you move forward in your nursing education, embrace these challenges with the knowledge that each effort you make is literally reshaping your brain and expanding your capabilities.

In Part I "Foundation for Thinking and Learning in Nursing School" you've gained insights into critical thinking, brain-based learning, and neuroplasticity. Understanding these fundamental concepts—the "how" and "why" of learning—provides you with an ability to apply your critical thinking to the content and strategies.

In Part II "Toolkit for Nursing School Success" you'll learn strategies for managing your thinking, time, lifestyle, stress, and anxiety, as well as how to leverage AI to enhance your learning. Use your critical thinking as you consider how the strategies align with brain-based learning and how neuroplasticity works in your favor. Let's begin with Chap. 4, where we'll delve into managing your thinking, which is essential for your academic and professional success.

> **Chapter 3 Synthesis Learning Activity: Boost Your Growth Mindset**
>
> This activity is designed to help you apply the growth mindset strategies you learned about in this chapter.
>
> 1. Describe how you would apply a growth mindset when you've just received a low grade on a nursing exam.
> 2. Identify an area in your nursing school experience where you tend to have a fixed mindset. This may be a course, or an assignment, or a component of courses like clinical experiences.

(continued)

(a) What are factors that influence your fixed mindset with this experience?

(b) List three strategies from the Practical Strategies list that you can apply as you work to shift from a fixed to a growth mindset with this experience.

3. Create a personal growth mindset mantra or affirmation that you can use when you face challenges in nursing school. Explain why you chose this mantra and how it embodies the principles of neuroplasticity and growth mindset.

References

Dweck, C. S. (2006). *Mindset: The new psychology of success*. Random House.

Gage, F. H. (2002). Neurogenesis in the adult brain. *Journal of Neuroscience, 22*(3), 612–613. https://doi.org/10.1523/JNEUROSCI.22-03-00612.2002

Hebb, D. O. (2002). The organization of behavior: A neuropsychological theory. *Psychology Press*. https://doi.org/10.4324/9781410612403

Jeffs, C., Nelson, N., Grant, K. A., Nowell, L., Paris, B., & Viceer, N. (2021). Feedback for teaching development: Moving from a fixed to growth mindset. *Professional Development in Education, 49*(5), 842–855. https://doi.org/10.1080/19415257.2021.1876149

Kolb, B. (2013). *Brain plasticity and behavior*. Psychology Press.

Lewis, L. S., Williams, C. A., & Dawson, S. (2024). Online mindset training for prelicensure nursing students: A randomized longitudinal study. *SAGE Open Nursing, 10*, 23779608241236285.

Williams, C. A. (2018). Mindsets may matter in nursing education. *Nursing Education Perspectives, 39*(6), 373–374. https://doi.org/10.1097/01.NEP.0000000000000267

Williams, C. A. (2020). Nursing students' mindsets matter: Cultivating a growth mindset. *Nurse Educator, 45*(5), 252–256. https://doi.org/10.1097/NNE.0000000000000798

Part II

Toolkit for Nursing School Success

Manage Your Thinking

4

Whether you think you can, or you think you can't—you're right.

—Henry Ford

4.1 Introduction

Managing your thoughts is the secret to nursing school success. As you begin your clinical courses, you're discovering that nursing school is challenging. This chapter explores how your self-talk—the ongoing conversation you have with yourself—affects your ability to learn, focus, and perform in class, clinical, and on exams. You'll discover why paying attention to your thoughts matters and learn practical strategies to keep your thinking positive and productive. Developing healthy thinking habits now will help you build a mindset that will serve you not just in nursing school, but throughout your nursing career.

▶ **By the end of this chapter you will be able to:**
1. Identify patterns of negative self-talk common in nursing students.
2. Understand the impact of self-talk on learning.
3. Develop techniques to interrupt negative thought patterns and replace them with positive self-talk affirmations.
4. Apply mindfulness practices and relaxation techniques to enhance focus and reduce stress during study sessions and clinical rotations.
5. Create a personalized plan for managing thoughts and relaxing your mind to optimize your academic performance and overall well-being in nursing school.

4.2 The Challenge of Thought Management in Nursing School

It's no secret—nursing school is hard!

To be successful in nursing school you need to:

- Comprehend what you are learning.
- Store learned information in long-term memory.
- Integrate new information with previously learned material.
- Apply learning to new and related situations that occur in clinical settings.

© The Author(s), under exclusive license to Springer Nature Switzerland AG 2025
C. Thompson, *Nursing School, NCLEX and Career Transition Success*,
https://doi.org/10.1007/978-3-031-85538-2_4

- Maximize learning in class, simulation, and clinical.
- Focus while you study.
- Focus during test taking.

And, you need to perform these functions quickly and accurately, which can be more challenging than anything you've experienced before. All of this pressure and intensity can bring your thoughts to a constant swirl and impact your ability to succeed.

As you learned in Chap. 3, adopting a growth mindset is essential for nursing school, helping you focus on learning and growth rather than just completing tasks. However, managing your thinking goes beyond adopting a growth mindset; it involves actively monitoring and controlling your self-talk, embracing positive thinking, and using mental techniques to enhance focus and reduce anxiety.

4.3 Understanding Self-Talk

Self-talk is the internal dialogue that runs through your mind throughout the day. It can be positive or negative, and it significantly impacts your motivation, confidence, and overall mental state. Our understanding that negative self-talk can create self-doubt and increase anxiety, while positive self-talk can enhance your confidence and reduce stress is not new (Beck, 1976).

Think about a time in your life when positive self-talk helped you succeed and a time when negative self-talk held you back. Your life experience will illuminate for you the impact of this relationship. The relationship between self-talk and outcomes is a strong and powerful association. In this chapter, you will identify your self-talk habits, and learn skills to turn your negative self-talk into positive.

Negative self-talk is associated with stress that leads to fight or flight response and reduces your brain's ability to focus, learn and retrieve previously learned information. On the other hand, positive self-talk optimizes your brain's capacity to learn, integrate, and apply information. Addressing self-talk is foundational to learning

and success in nursing school and to your overall well-being (Xiao et al., 2023).

4.3.1 Why Is Self-Talk Difficult to Manage?

Your brain processes patterns. The more a thought pattern is repeated, the more automatic it becomes. Let's think back to the time in your life when you can recall a relationship between positive self-talk and outcomes. As you reflect on that time, can you see that you were strongly embedded in the positive thinking. On the other hand, as you reflect on a time you were in a slump, you may recall how difficult it was to get yourself out of that slump. Your brain was processing those patterns of self-talk on repeat.

In nursing school, allowing negative self-talk to go unchecked keeps the thoughts on repeat. Your brain and body are flooded with stress hormones that you can literally become addicted to. This is one reason why changing negative self-talk can be challenging (Carroll, 2022).

4.3.2 Positive and Negative Self-Talk

Table 4.1 contrasts negative and positive self-talk in nursing school.

There are multiple impacts of self-talk that have been reported by many authors (Alicke & Sedikides, 2010; Dweck, 2006; Kim et al., 2021). Negative self-talk impacts your ability to think, focus, learn, and be creative (Kross et al., 2014). Let's look in more detail at these factors associated with self-talk so you can better understand how self-talk influences your ability to be positive, think clearly, learn, and apply critical thinking.

Neuroplasticity as you recall is the brain's ability to reorganize and form new neural connections in response to learning experiences. The habit of negative self-talk creates pathways that perpetuate negative thoughts. On the other hand, positive self-talk creates pathways that lead to more positive thoughts.

4.3 Understanding Self-Talk

Table 4.1 Negative versus positive self-talk

Negative self-talk	Positive self-talk
This is too much to learn	I am grateful to learn and grow
I know I'm going to fail this test	I know this test is going to be hard but I am prepared and will do my best
I probably did that wrong because I always get nervous in clinical situations and make mistakes	I am here to learn. I will improve with practice
I don't raise my hand in class because I will say the wrong thing	Participating in class helps me learn even if my answers aren't always correct
I don't learn anything when we have a flipped class	Flipped classes are hard for me but they help me engage in brain-based learning
I can't learn anything from that instructor	I am not a fan of that instructor's teaching but I will adapt to get the most out of the course
I study hard but always end up studying the wrong things	I use my critical thinking skills to identify key concepts to link my understanding
I study hard but don't learn what the instructor wants me to know	I adapt my studying to my learning style to better understand what I am learning

Stress response is activated by negative self-talk and triggers release of stress hormones like cortisol, which can disrupt neurotransmitter balance in the brain and impairs memory, attention, and decision-making.

Attention is diverted by negative thoughts from the task at hand making it difficult to concentrate and engage in critical thinking.

Learning capacity is diminished by negative self-talk because it reinforces rigid thinking patterns. This limits the ability to focus, learn information, and recall learned information. Like neuroplasticity, positive self-talk has the opposite impact, increasing capacity to focus, learning, and information recall.

Cognitive Flexibility refers to the ability to adapt thinking to new situations. Negative self-talk makes it harder to consider different perspectives or change approaches when needed. Positive self-talk expands capacity for openness.

Confidence, a key aspect of critical thinking, is eroded by negative self-talk. Constant self-doubt makes it harder to trust one's own judgment and make decisions whereas positive self-talk builds confidence.

Creativity is stifled by negative self-talk because it increases fear of judgment or failure. This reduces the likelihood of thinking outside the box or proposing innovative ideas.

Self-Efficacy is the belief in one's ability to succeed in specific situations. Negative self-talk weakens this belief, making a person feel less capable of handling challenges or solving problems effectively whereas positive self-talk improves your belief in your abilities.

Positive self-talk creates a neurobiological environment that facilitates formation of new neural pathways, enhancing integration of new knowledge and skills. Reduced stress levels that occur with positive thinking improves focus and attention and facilitates your ability to learn, process, integrate, and apply new information to previously learned information. This fosters a growth mindset, which you learned in the previous chapter is essential for effective learning and critical thinking.

Complete Self-Assessment 4.1 to review your self-talk patterns.

Self-Assessment 4.1: Self-Talk

The purpose of this self-assessment is for you to note your self-talk. Pay attention to and record your self-talk during three different nursing school-related activities; studying for an exam, receiving feedback from an instructor and during a class session.

Record your self-talk statements in Table 4.2 Self-Talk Record, then mark in the appropriate column if each statement was a negative or positive self–talk statement.

Consider each of the following questions as you reflect on your self-talk.

Table 4.2 Self-talk record

Studying for class or an exam	Negative	Positive

Receiving feedback from an instructor	Negative	Positive

During a class session	Negative	Positive

1. What is the frequency of your negative thoughts?
2. In which circumstances is your self-talk more negative than positive?
3. Are there recurring themes in your self-talk such as fear of failure, or lack of confidence?
4. What relationship can you see between your self-talk and your performance?

It is important to catch your negative thoughts, interrupt them, and substitute positive self-talk. This is referred to as thought monitoring.

Correcting negative self-talk involves metacognitive processes such as self-awareness and self-regulation. By monitoring and challenging your thoughts, you develop a deeper understanding of your learning process and become more adept at evaluating and adjusting your thinking strategies.

Understanding why and how self-talk supports your ability to learn should increase your motivation to adopt positive self-talk. Replacing negative self-talk with positive affirmation will improve your learning and critical thinking.

4.4 📝 Practical Strategies: Managing Self-Talk

Now that you've assessed your self-talk patterns and reflected on their impact, let's explore some practical strategies to help you cultivate more positive self-talk and manage your thinking effectively. These techniques will help you transform negative thought patterns into supportive, growth-oriented self-dialogue that enhances your learning and performance in nursing school.

- **Create a positive self-talk mantra**

The mantra should be words that feel right for you. This should be a broad statement that you can use regularly to transform your mindset. Sample mantras include:

"I will be a nurse."
"I can conquer nursing school."
"I am strong."
"I am smart."

- **Use your self-talk mantra on a regular basis**

The more you repeat your self-talk mantra, the more likely you are to adopt it and support your growth mindset. You could:

(a) Repeat your mantra every morning.
(b) Write your mantra on your bathroom mirror.
(c) Place your mantra on a sticky note on your computer.
(d) Incorporate your mantra into a daily morning meditation routine.

- **Stop negative self-talk**

Find a strategy that works for you and use that every time you have a negative thought. Use a STOP strategy and replace the negative with positive. Some evidence-based examples for interrupting negative thoughts include:

(a) Wear an elastic band on your wrist and gently snap it.
(b) Take 4-7-8 breaths (4 s inhale, 7 s hold, 8 s exhale).
(c) Rotate your head side to side and say "no" to the negative thought.
(d) Envision your negative thoughts floating off to the sky in a thought bubble that pops, with the words becoming invisible when the bubble pops.
(e) Imagine your hands pulling the negative thoughts out of your head.

- **Practice positive thought imagery**

When you find yourself spiraling into negative thoughts or feeling overwhelmed, try a simple imagery exercise to redirect your focus to help you transition back to positive thinking. For example:

(a) Immerse yourself in thoughts of your special relaxing and happy place; at the beach, in the mountains, on your best vacation.
(b) Create an image of yourself on your last day of class for the semester, you've checked your grades and you've performed well.
(c) Imagine your graduation day, you are surrounded by your friends and family and everyone is happy for you.
(d) Picture yourself in your scrubs with your name followed by RN on your name badge.

- **Surround yourself with peers who also practice positive self-talk**

You don't have to look far in nursing school to find classmates who verbalize their negative thoughts and work to bring others into that thinking. If you find yourself surrounded by peers who complain about instructors, assignments, class activities, clinical sites, exam questions or anything that comes along, or who project overall negativity "I know we are all going to fail" distance yourself from those individuals.

You may not be able to physically do this. You find yourself in a clinical group with a group of students who frequently complain. You can't leave the group, but you can pay attention to your thoughts and be intentional about recognizing the negative patterns of the thoughts your group members share.

Now that you understand the impact of negative self-talk on your critical thinking and learning, if you tend toward negative self-talk, you can commit to adopting strategies to make positivity the language of your thoughts.

4.5 Relaxing Your Mind

Another crucial aspect of managing your thoughts is relaxing your mind. While self-talk influences your internal dialogue, mind relaxation techniques help create a calm mental environment that supports critical thinking and learning. Just as positive self-talk can rewire your brain for success, regular mind relaxation practices can enhance your ability to focus, retain information, and apply your knowledge effectively (Benson & Proctor, 2011).

There is little in our culture that supports mind relaxation. Multitasking, constant activity, and overcommitment have become normalized even though we know it does not improve our ability to learn and be productive (Garner & Dux, 2023). With constant access to an "online" world, and demands for multitasking, anxiety, depression, and other mental health disorders have surged and studies have demonstrated associations between excessive social media use and various mental health concerns, including anxiety, depression, and other psychological disorders (Karim et al., 2020; Zubair et al., 2023). From a neurophysiological perspective, our brains have not evolved to adapt to this change and as a result, we accept the erosion of our well-being while we adapt to the demands of society.

Brain overstimulation that happens as a routine part of our day-to-day life leads to stress and the release of stress hormones like epinephrine. The stress response provides a physiological mechanism that enables us to react to immediate threats, such as encountering a bear. During this response, heart rate increases to supply oxygen to muscles, pupils dilate to enhance vision, and blood is redirected to essential organs for survival. Our brain's focus narrows to prioritize survival instincts. Once the threat passes, our body returns to a balanced state of homeostasis.

Repeated activation of the stress response creates a chronic state of arousal, which is where most of us live on a day-to-day basis. From this heightened state of arousal, we can then tip more easily to full blown panic.

It is difficult to perform your best academically when you are living in the constant state of brain arousal. Under chronic stress, the brain's prefrontal cortex, responsible for higher-order functions such as problem-solving, decision making, and critical thinking, becomes less effective. At the same time, the amygdala, which processes emotions, especially fear, becomes more reactive. This imbalance can lead to difficulties in concentration, memory retention, and learning new information (McEwen et al., 2015).

By contrast, when the mind is relaxed, the brain can function optimally. In a calm state, the prefrontal cortex can perform at its best, allowing for improved focus, enhanced memory, and better problem-solving abilities. Mind relaxation activities enhance neuroplasticity, which helps your brain form new neural connections. The calm state that is induced by relaxation decreases production of stress hormones, which improves attention and focus. Regular mind relaxation also changes the density of gray meeting in the regions of the brain associated with learning, memory, and emotional regulation (Davidson & McEwen, 2012).

You can see the link between these brain neurophysiological changes and brain-based learning. Mind relaxation creates an environment where the brain can operate in a balanced state to optimize your academic success, while also improving your overall well-being.

Now that you understand the basics of why mind relaxation is important, complete the Mind Relaxation Self-Assessment to determine where you are and then consider ways you can improve.

Self-Assessment 4.2: Mind Relaxation

Relaxing your mind is essential for effective learning and overall well-being. In a constantly connected world, managing distractions and cultivating mindfulness can significantly impact your academic performance and mental health. This self-assessment will help you evaluate your current habits and identify areas where you can improve your practices to ensure your mind is relaxed and focused. By developing better relaxation techniques and minimizing distractions, you can enhance your ability to absorb and retain information, leading to greater success in your studies and future nursing career.

Answer each of the following questions in Table 4.3 to assess your current mind relaxation habits:

If you answered "Yes" to most of these questions:

You have already committed to practices that help you relax your mind. Even when you are busy, recognize the importance of your practices as essential for your learning.

If you answered "No" to many of these questions:

You can make simple changes that will substantially improve your capacity for brain-based learning and critical thinking. Review the Practical Strategies and now that you understand the importance of mind relaxation, try out different ones to find what works best for you. Then commit to that practice.

Developing effective mind relaxation habits is an ongoing process. Be patient with yourself as you work to incorporate these practices into your routine. Even small improvements can lead to significant benefits in your learning and overall well-being as a nursing student.

Table 4.3 Self-assessment mind relaxation

Mind relaxation	Yes	No
When I am studying, I silence my phone and disconnect notifications on my watch to avoid distraction		
When I am studying I avoid scrolling through social media		
When in class I silence my phone away and disconnect notifications on my watch so that I am not distracted		
When I am in class I avoid scrolling through social media		
I am mindful about my learning; when I study I focus on the content I am learning and avoid distracting thoughts such as "will this be on the test?"		
I have a practice (yoga, journaling, prayer, mindfulness) to relax my mind that I use on a regular basis		
I practice gratitude on a regular basis		
When I find myself multi-tasking I bring an awareness to stop		
I have taken steps to reduce my nonessential screen time		
I am mindful while I eat; I sit down and focus on the food I am eating, how it tastes and how it is filling me, instead of looking at my device or multitasking		
I cultivate a positive mindset to help me stay focused		

Nursing School Application: Relaxed Mind Approach to Exam Preparation

Now that we've explored the theoretical aspects of managing thinking and mind relaxation, let's see how these concepts can be applied in a real-world nursing school scenario. The following example illustrates how a student, Skylar, uses relaxation techniques and positive self-talk to prepare for and succeed in a crucial exam. After examining this practical application, we'll delve into specific strategies you can adopt to relax your mind and enhance your learning experience.

Skylar's course exam average is 0.5% points above passing the course. This scenario takes place the evening before the third of four course exams.

Skylar has adopted a practice of morning gratitude and journaling that she has found keeps her grounded throughout nursing school. Just like every other nursing student, she can get caught up in anxiety and deadlines and worry, but she uses her practice to keep her at a low stress baseline and commits to the practice even when she is busy because she recognizes the degree to which it helps her. As part of her gratitude, she reminds herself that her hard work (this upcoming test that she has to really commit to studying for) contributes to her goal of becoming a nurse. It has been her dream since elementary school.

Skylar knows her exam average is on the borderline but reminds herself that she has been in this circumstance before and has done better in the second half of her courses when she knows more about how the what will be emphasized on the tests. Skylar begins her study time with a few deep breaths to bring her heart rate and breathing down and focus her on studying. She closes her eyes and envisions this exam grade displayed on her computer—85%. This is well above what she needs to pass the course.

During her study time, Skylar links information from the previous learning and writes notes about those connections. At 8 PM Skylar completed the pre-class reading, listened to the online lecture, and wrote notes on key points. Skylar decides to go for a short run, then come back and hang out with friends before going to bed at 11 PM. She falls asleep within 10 min of lying down and sleeps until 6:30 AM.

Before the exam, Skylar takes a few deep breaths and reminds herself that she is well prepared. She stays focused throughout the exam and scores 84.5%. This grade brings her exam average up and out of the danger zone. Skylar is confident she will do well on her fourth and final course exam.

Skylar's approach demonstrates how effectively managing thoughts and incorporating relaxation techniques can positively impact performance. Her success isn't just luck—it's the result of deliberate practices that support a relaxed, focused mind. Let's explore specific strategies you can implement to achieve similar results in your nursing school journey.

4.6   📝 Practical Strategies: Mind Relaxation

Now that you understand the importance of mind relaxation for your learning, let's explore specific strategies to help you. If you're new to mind relaxation practices, be patient with yourself as you experiment to find which strategies work for you. Remember, you're essentially rewiring your brain during this transition, which takes time and persistence.

These strategies share a common goal: to quiet the constant chatter and busy work of your mind. The state of calm you can achieve will reset your brain's neurophysiologic homeostasis.

As you work on these practices you'll notice improvements in your ability to manage stress, stay focused, learn, retain information, and perform at your best in your nursing studies. The benefits extend beyond academics, contributing to your overall well-being and preparing you for the demands of your future nursing career.

- **Adopt a daily practice for relaxing your mind and commit to it for at least 15 min per day**

Activities to relax your mind that include meditation, prayer, yoga, or journaling as examples. The important element of each of these is creating time where you quiet your mind. Committed meditative practice actually changes the structure of your brain, opening processing pathways that are inhibited by constant mind chatter.

This is one of the easiest strategies to enhance your learning. Perhaps you already have a daily practice. It will be easier to stick with it now that you understand "why" it is important and "how" it helps your learning.

If you do not have a committed practice, beginning will be difficult at first. This is because your brain chatter is like an addiction; when you try to stop it, your brain will give you intense urgency to keep it up. You may find it helpful to begin in small increments; begin with a 5 min practice, then increase your time.

Whatever you choose for a relaxation practice, you can find free and low cost apps available to assist you on this journey.

- **Be mindful in your learning**

You may have learned about the importance of mindfulness for reducing stress and improving your overall well-being. Being mindful in your learning in nursing school supports your thought management.

Short bursts of mindfulness with self-affirmation have been linked to brain changes that improve processing (Cohen & Sherman, 2014; Luo et al., 2024). You can adopt a mindful minute to refocus before class, study sessions, working on an assignment or a clinical day. A "mindful minute" practice looks like this:

Close your eyes. Take a deep calming breath. Repeat to yourself appropriate mindful minute statements. Some examples include saying before class:

"I am here to learn."
"My mind is clear."
"I am ready to absorb the information that will be covered."
"This is where I learn on my journey to become a nurse."
"Here is where I will apply what I have learned."
"I have the ability to understand what I am studying."

- **Practice gratitude**

Gratitude is another practice that not only improves well-being but enhances learning. One fundamental gratitude practice that is easy to overlook when you are in the hectic pace of nursing school is acknowledging how fortunate you are to be in nursing school.

In 2023, over 70,000 qualified applicants were not accepted to nursing schools in the United States (AACN, 2024). You are fortunate to be able to pursue your dream. Many others didn't even get the chance to begin!

This is one strategy to enhance your learning. Take time each morning, or before a class, to make a mental or written list of things you are grateful for.

- **Manage your stress**

It is well documented that nursing is one of the most stressful academic programs. The competition, the pressure to pass exams and progress to the next course, performing in clinical and simulation experiences, high stakes testing, hearing classmates talk about stress, all of these things add to the mix of stress. There are plenty of nursing students who started nursing school as happy, calm, well-balanced individuals who by the end were a bundle of nerves.

Stress is detrimental in so many ways and as noted in the previous section, is a negative self-talk trigger. Stress management is key to your well-being and to your academic success. More on this topic is included in Chap. 7.

- **Limit your screen time**

Screen time provides intense brain stimulation. Even when you use blue light blocking lenses or filters, screens stimulate your brain. For many of us, screen time has replaced quiet time. When you arrive in your nursing classroom what do you see? Students on devices instead of talking to each other.

Much of your nursing school work requires screen time. Because you will not be able to eliminate that screen time you can help your brain by cutting down on nonessential screen time.

Taking a break from screen time lets your brain rest and recharge, which improves your focus, concentration, ability to learn, and overall well-being.

- **Evaluate and reduce your social media activity**

You've heard it said social media is an addiction, and you may have even become aware of that and tried to make changes for yourself.

When you check your social media and there's a message or video for you a surge of dopamine is released and that makes your brain feel good. It's why we are frequently moved to check in on our social media accounts. Your brain wants that dopamine, which propels your addiction and overrides whatever else you are processing in your brain. This is why it is so difficult for anyone to give up their social media.

Consider setting limits on your social media while you are in nursing school. Who knows, you may like being less distracted and decide not to resume your social media even after you've graduated and begun your nursing career.

- **Practice deep breathing**

You can't simultaneously activate your parasympathetic (calm) and sympathetic (stress) nervous systems. Focusing on a slow deep breath engages your parasympathetic nervous system, which helps your body relax and your mind become calm.

Try it: take a 4–7-8 breath. Inhale deeply for 4 s, hold for 7 s, and exhale slowly for 8 s. Can you feel the calm settling in?

Just like 1 min mindfulness, this deep breathing technique is one you can use to calm your mind before class, during an exam, or before a study session. As you begin to practice using deep breathing, you will find that you can more easily regulate calmness to relax your mind.

4.7 Conclusion

In this chapter, we explored strategies to manage your thinking and demonstrated the relationship between these strategies and brain neurophysiology, helping you understand how and why positive self-talk and mind relaxation are important for your success. By embracing positive thinking and using mental techniques to relax your mind you can be more successful in nursing school. These strategies are part of broader lifestyle practices that support critical thinking by optimizing brain-based learning. They are not only useful during your time in nursing school but will also serve you well in your nursing practice and life in general.

In the next chapter we turn our attention to another crucial aspect of nursing school success: time management. Just as a relaxed and focused mind enhances your learning, efficient use of your time can significantly boost your productivity and reduce stress.

Chapter 4: Synthesis Learning Activity: Mastering Your Mental Landscape

This activity is designed to help you apply the concepts learned in this chapter to your own thought patterns and stress responses. By transforming negative self-talk and developing strategies for managing stress, you'll create a personalized toolkit for maintaining a positive mindset throughout your nursing education.

1. Self-Talk Transformation:
   (a) Identify three negative self-talk statements you frequently use.
   (b) Rewrite each statement as a positive, growth-oriented affirmation.
   (c) Create a plan to incorporate these new affirmations into your daily routine.
2. Stress Scenario Response:
   Imagine you have three exams and a clinical evaluation in the same week. Write a step-by-step plan using both positive self-talk and mind relaxation strategies to manage this stressful situation.
3. Learning Environment Audit:
   List three changes you can make in your primary study space to create a more relaxed, focused environment.

Mastering your mental well-being is an ongoing process. By completing this activity, you'll develop practical skills for managing your thoughts and stress responses. Regularly reflect on these practices and adjust them as needed to support your growth and success in nursing school.

References

Alicke, M. D., & Sedikides, C. (2010). *Handbook of self-enhancement and self-protection*. Guilford Publications.

American Association of Colleges of Nursing (AACN). (2024, May). *Nursing faculty shortage fact sheet*. Retrieved November 7, 2024 from https://www.aacnnursing.org/news-data/fact-sheets/nursing-faculty-shortage

Beck, A. T. (1976). *Cognitive therapy and the emotional disorders*. Penguin.

Benson, H., & Proctor, W. (2011). *Relaxation revolution: The science and genetics of mind body healing*. Simon and Schuster.

Carroll, A. (2022). *The impact of self-talk on college students' self-esteem, educational self-efficacy, and mood*. Doctoral dissertation. Dublin: National College of Ireland.

Cohen, G., & Sherman, D. (2014). The psychology of change: Self-affirmation and social psychological intervention. *Annual Review of Psychology, 65*, 333–371. https://doi.org/10.1146/annurev-psych-010213-115137

Davidson, R. J., & McEwen, B. S. (2012). Social influences on neuroplasticity: Stress and interventions to promote well-being. *Nature Neuroscience, 15*(5), 689–695.

Dweck, C. S. (2006). *Mindset: The new psychology of success*. Random House.

Garner, K. G., & Dux, P. E. (2023). Knowledge generalization and the costs of multitasking. *Nature Reviews Neuroscience, 24*(2), 98–112. https://doi.org/10.1038/s41583-022-00653-x

Karim, F., Oyewande, A. A., Abdalla, L. F., Chaudhry Ehsanullah, R., & Khan, S. (2020). Social media use and its connection to mental health: A systematic review. *Cureus, 12*(6), e8627. https://doi.org/10.7759/cureus.8627

Kim, J., Kwon, J. H., Kim, J., Kim, E. J., Kim, H. E., Kyeong, S., & Kim, J. J. (2021). The effects of positive or negative self-talk on the alteration of brain functional connectivity by performing cognitive tasks. *Scientific Reports, 11*(1), 14873. https://doi.org/10.1038/s41598-021-94328-9

Kross, E., Bruehlman-Senecal, E., Park, J., Burson, A., Dougherty, A., Shablack, H., Bremner, R., Moser, J., & Ayduk, O. (2014). Self-talk as a regulatory mechanism: How you do it matters. *Journal of Personality and Social Psychology, 106*(2), 304–324. https://doi.org/10.1037/a0035173

Luo, J., Cao, J., Yeung, P., Ng, J., & Sun, M. (2024). Mindfulness and growth mindset as protective factors for the impact of media multitasking on academic performance: The mediating role of self-control. *Education and Information Technologies.* https://doi.org/10.1007/s10639-024-12759-z

McEwen, B. S., Bowles, N. P., Gray, J. D., Hill, M. N., Hunter, R. G., Karatsoreos, I. N., & Nasca, C. (2015). Mechanisms of stress in the brain. *Nature Neuroscience, 18*(10), 1353–1363.

Xiao, F., Zhang, Z., Zhou, J., Wu, H., Zhang, L., Lin, M., & Hu, L. (2023). The relationship between a growth mindset and the learning engagement of nursing students: A structural equation modeling approach. *Nurse Education in Practice, 73*, 103796. https://doi.org/10.1016/j.nepr.2023.103796

Zubair, U., Khan, M. K., & Albashari, M. (2023). Link between excessive social media use and psychiatric disorders. *Annals of Medicine and Surgery, 85*(4), 875–878. https://doi.org/10.1097/MS9.0000000000000112

Manage Your Time

5

The bad news is time flies. The good news is you're the pilot.

—Michael Altshuler

5.1   Introduction

You've made it this far in nursing school, which means you already have some grasp on managing your time. But let's face it—nursing school takes time management to a whole new level. The demands are intense, the material is complex, and the stakes are high. This chapter will help you refine your time management skills specifically for nursing school success. By the end of this chapter, you'll have the tools to take control of your schedule so you can make your way through nursing school with less stress and more success.

▶ **By the end of this chapter you will be able to:**
1. Analyze time management.
2. Identify time-wasters and distractions.
3. Create a schedule to balance study time, self-care, and other responsibilities.
4. Maximize productive hours and make the most of short time blocks.
5. Build rest and recovery time into time management scheduling to support learning and well-being.

5.2   Nursing School Time Management

Have you ever found yourself frantically cramming for an exam at 2 AM, wondering where all your study time went? Or perhaps you've had to choose between finishing an assignment and getting enough sleep? Maybe you've missed out on important family events or self-care time because schoolwork always seems to take priority? If any of this sounds familiar, you're not alone.

Being constantly busy isn't just exhausting, it's counterproductive to learning. Yet most nursing students find themselves with a to-do list that's longer than their available hours in the day.

As you learned in Part I of this book, brain-based learning, adopting a growth mindset and using critical thinking are critical to your nursing school, NCLEX, and nursing practice success. The right mix of learning, self-care, and sleep to process and integrate new information is essential for your success.

© The Author(s), under exclusive license to Springer Nature Switzerland AG 2025
C. Thompson, *Nursing School, NCLEX and Career Transition Success*,
https://doi.org/10.1007/978-3-031-85538-2_5

When we take a closer look at our daily routines, we often discover that much of our "free" time isn't truly restful or productive. Scrolling social media, binge-watching shows, or even just worrying about all we have to do are activities that don't recharge us or move us forward.

Effective time management isn't about squeezing more tasks into your day. It's about making intentional choices that align with your priorities and support your success.

Before we dive into strategies for better time management, it's crucial to have a clear picture of where your time is actually going. You might be surprised by what you discover! Many students find they're spending more time on certain activities than they realized, or that they're not using their most productive hours effectively.

Complete the Time Management Self-Assessment 5.1 to begin the process of evaluating ways to improve your time management.

Self-Assessment 5.1: Time Management

A time study is an analysis of your daily time flow. When you review your time management record, you can use critical thinking to help you see how to improve your time management.

Record your hourly time activities.

Unless you are in an online nursing program, most likely you have a pattern in which your Monday–Friday schedule includes classes and clinical. For your time study, it will be helpful for you to record your hourly activity on a typical weekday (Table 5.1) and again for a typical weekend day (Table 5.2).

Now that you have a record of your activities that you can review, complete the Self-Assessment 5.2 to outline our time management needs.

Table 5.1 Weekday activity record

Date of recording activity for a weekday _____ _____

Time	Activity	Had to do	Wanted to do	Did not need to do
6–7 am				
7–8 am				
8–9 am				
9–10 am				
10–11 am				
11–12 pm				
12–1 pm				
1–2 pm				
2–3 pm				
3–4 pm				
4–5 pm				
5–6 pm				
6–7 pm				
7–8 pm				
8–9 pm				
9–10 pm				
10–11 pm				

Table 5.2 Weekend day activity record

Date of recording activity for a weekend day _____ _____

Time	Activity	Had to do	Wanted to do	Did not need to do
6–7 am				
7–8 am				
8–9 am				
9–10 am				
10–11 am				
11–12 pm				
12–1 pm				
1–2 pm				
2–3 pm				
3–4 pm				
4–5 pm				
5–6 pm				
6–7 pm				
7–8 pm				
8–9 pm				
9–10 pm				
10–11 pm				

5.2 Nursing School Time Management

Self-Assessment 5.2: Time Management Needs

Analyzing how you spend your time is a crucial step in improving time management. By applying critical thinking to your time record, you can identify areas for improvement and make changes that will enhance your learning and overall nursing school experience.
Begin your analysis by having you categorize your time activity needs in Table 5.3.

Go back to Tables 5.1 and 5.2 and mark your most productive times.

When are your peak productivity times?
Weekday _____
Weekend _____

Review your time records and list three activities that you feel were not productive uses of your time.

1. _____
2. _____
3. _____

Review your time record and identify where you felt rushed and unable to complete what you needed with a growth mindset.

Review your time record and identify where you spent too much time being unproductive in a way that did not support your overall well-being.

Reflect on the following question: How well does my current time allocation align with my priorities and goals?

Write two to three specific changes you could make to improve your time management to optimize your critical thinking, brain-based learning, and growth mindset?

Your time management self-assessment may help you determine a structure for time management that will work best for you. There are various ways to accomplish this.

Table 5.3 Category time assessment

Category	Weekday hours	Weekend hours	Total hours
Sleep			
Class			
Study			
Work			
Family			
Leisure			
Self-care			
Other			

Now that you've gained insights into your current time management habits, it's time to put that knowledge into action. You've identified your peak productivity times, recognized potential time-wasters, and reflected on how well your current schedule aligns with your goals. This self-awareness is a powerful tool, but it's just the first step.

The next challenge is to translate these insights into a schedule that supports your learning and well-being. Creating a schedule isn't about forcing yourself into a rigid routine. Instead, it's about applying your critical thinking to design a schedule that maximizes your productivity during your best hours, minimizes time-wasters, and ensures a balance between study, work, and self-care.

In the following section, we'll explore different approaches to creating an effective schedule. There is not a one-size-fits-all solution. The goal is to find a method that works for you. As you review the strategies, consider how they might address challenges you identified in your self-assessment.

5.2.1 Creating an Effective Schedule

Just like a budget helps you manage your money, a schedule will help you manage your time and boost your brain-based learning. There are several strategies for creating a schedule.

5.2.1.1 Semester or Term Schedule

You have probably already discovered that your schedule for nursing school is rigorous. An essential time management strategy is to create an overview of your time needs for each semester or term. You can do this when you get the syllabus for each of the courses you are taking.

When you overview your semester or term, you will see there will be weeks that are more demanding than others. Most courses are laid out with about four major exams. One of these may be a midterm exam, and one may be a final exam. If you are taking more than one nursing course, these exams may be in the same week.

With this in mind, creating a schedule for each week that incorporates time for study and review of content will support your ability to be prepared for those weeks with multiple exams and assignments.

5.2.1.2 Daily or Weekly Schedule

It is well established that writing a schedule helps you stay organized and productive with time management. You may already have a strategy that works for you. Here are two examples of scheduling that you could consider.

Calendar Schedule with Time Blocking

A detailed calendar that outlines your activity for each day is the most structured format for managing time. You create your schedule for each day, based on your class, clinical, work and schedule for other responsibilities. You can create this schedule in a written planner or using an online tool.

This format is similar to hours recording in the time study you completed. While this may take more time to lay out, you may find it easier to follow when your schedule does not allow for wiggle room.

If you tend to procrastinate you may find that a detailed schedule will work best. As you create your schedule, be sure it is feasible so that you can stick to it.

When you block time, you create a task list for time intervals for each day. Table 5.4 outlines a weekday block time schedule.

This tool allows you to create a schedule for each day. You can lay out this format for a week, or at the end of the day create your time block for the next day.

Table 5.4 Time blocking

Time	Activity
7:15–7:30	Mind relaxing
7:30–8	Review for class
8–10	Classes
10:10–11	Study
11–12	Lunch
12–1	Review for class
1–3	Classes
3:10–4:00	Study
4–5	Errands
5–6	Physical activity
6–6:30	Dinner
6:30–8:30	Studying
8:30–bed	Relaxing

Table 5.5 Task blocking

Class days		Clinical days		Weekend days	
Activity	Hours	Activity	Hours	Activity	Hours
Class	6	Clinical	9	Work	4
Study	4	Study	2	Study	4
Mind relaxing	0.5	Mind relaxing	0.5	Mind relaxing	0.5
Relax	2	Relax	1	Relax	4
Physical activity	1	Physical activity	0.5	Physical activity	
Other (eat, errands, travel)	1.5	Other	1.5	Other	2

Calendar Scheduling With Task Blocking

Another time scheduling option is to outline allotted times for activities. This allows you to create a schedule that you can use for your academic days and days "off" school. Table 5.5 outlines a task blocking calendar.

No matter what format you choose for organizing and managing your time, the purpose of time management is to support your ability to move through nursing school using brain-based learning. Maintaining a balance between coursework, outside commitments, and downtime is crucial for your well-being.

5.3 📋 Practical Strategies: Working During Nursing School

For many nursing students, there's a significant factor that complicates this balance: work. Financial needs often make working during nursing school not just common, but necessary. While employment can provide essential financial support and valuable experience, it also presents unique challenges to effective time management and learning.

This section explores strategies to manage work commitments without compromising your academic success or well-being. By understanding the impact of work on your brain-based learning and applying critical thinking to your work–study balance, you can use the same critical thinking skills you're developing for your studies.

For some students working a few hours each week is the right amount to have a distraction from nursing school while making ends meet. If this describes your work/nursing school balance, congratulations!

Working during school is the normal reality for most nursing students, and many find themselves in situations where work does interfere with their ability to apply a growth mindset throughout their learning. If you are not doing your best learning to support your critical thinking and your ability to think like a nurse, here are some things to reflect on and consider:

- **Avoid night shifts**

  Sleep is integral to brain-based learning, and for that reason, 6–8 h of uninterrupted sleep during the natural circadian cycle of sleep is best. Your individual circumstances may be such that you can't avoid night shift, however, if you do work night shift, this is a good time to consider other options that may better support your learning.

- **Balance full-time studies with work**

  Full-time student status is just that, full time. The expectation is your academic schedule should consume at least 40 h per week. If you are working another 36–40 h per week on top of your school schedule, you are compromising both your learning and your well-being. Even for the most capable students, balancing full-time work with full-time studies can be extremely challenging and may compromise your learning and well-being. Falling behind in a course due to a full-time work schedule risks course failure, which in the end is a high price to pay.

- **Prioritize sleep before class/clinical**

  You may believe you are herculean and you can work a night shift and then function through a day of activity. Perhaps you have done this for many years. Even if you believe missing a night of sleep does not impact your ability to function, the neurophysiology of learning tells us otherwise. You cannot safely provide care in clinical, nor can you optimize your learning when you approach either after a night of work.

- **Rethink your work hours**

  If your work commitments are causing you stress, surely you have considered other options. Revisit your big picture again and rethink strategies to reduce your work hours while you are in school. Create a detailed budget to identify areas where you can cut expenses, allowing you to potentially reduce work hours. Can you:

  - Decrease your spending?
  - Increase your work hours during semester breaks?
  - Increase your income during semester breaks?

  Sometimes we get into a routine of doing what we do, and don't stop to reconsider how important each thing is to our end goal. Taking time to review your goals and budget may help you identify opportunities for change.

- **Consider long-term costs**

  Not finding the right balance between work and school increases your risk for using a fixed mindset approach, shortcutting learning to complete assignments on time. This interferes with your ability to use brain-based learning, apply critical thinking, and build your foundation of learning.

The short-term impact of this approach is not passing a course. The long-term impact is not being prepared for NCLEX when you graduate. There are financial setbacks with either of these outcomes.

When you fail a course, in addition to paying to retake the course, you are delaying your timeline for reaching that nurse's paycheck.

Most nursing programs do not allow you to continue after a second course failure. Program dismissal due to course failure is devastating, leaving a student with school debt and no prospects for the income boost that comes with a job as a nurse to pay off that debt.

Not being prepared for NCLEX creates a challenge that leaves students without a safety net. When you graduate from your nursing program, you will be on your own for your final NCLEX preparation (see Chap. 13). Even though you will have an NCLEX preparation resource, filling in knowledge gaps that are cumulative is challenging. NCLEX failure is an even greater setback that can result in a job offer being rescinded. This further delays moving into a nursing position with a nurse's pay. In addition, NCLEX failure leads to a spiral for many graduates who do not pass on their first attempt. Repeat NCLEX pass rates are less than 50% (NCSBN, 2024). This is a circumstance that has devastating financial consequences.

While this outlines a grim scenario, one that you may not see yourself in, it is something to consider if your work schedule interferes with your ability to embrace a growth mindset. Use your critical thinking to decide if your work is upsetting the balance and putting you at risk for negative outcomes.

- **Prioritize self-care**

While balancing work and nursing school, it's crucial not to overlook self-care. Taking care of your mental and physical well-being is essential for effective brain-based learning.

Managing your time will help you become more organized and make the most of your learning in nursing school. You can prioritize the tasks needed, so you have leisure time without stress. Good time management results in improved brain-based learning; greater productivity, reduced stress, improved efficiency, and better critical thinking.

Balancing work and nursing school is a delicate act. Finding the right balance between work and school not only supports your current learning but also sets you up for success in your nursing career.

Nursing School Application: Time Management: A Tale of Two Students

Mala trying to do it all.

Mala entered nursing school with high hopes and determination to succeed. She knew she would have to maintain her full-time job during nursing school, but her work as a Patient Care Assistant in a busy Emergency Department (ED) inspired her to become an ED nurse. She worked with others who balanced work and school and enrolled in a nursing program that accommodated working students.

Determined to handle both full-time work and school, Mala switched to the night shift. As she began her nursing courses, Mala found herself constantly juggling assignments, work, and basic needs like sleep. She arrived at morning classes exhausted from her night shift. Though she managed to stay awake during classes, staying awake during her study time was a struggle. Her study sessions became sporadic, often squeezed into quiet moments during work or hurried attempts just before deadlines.

Mala's grades began to suffer. Even though she intended to embrace a growth mindset for her learning, she found herself

(continued)

spiraling into a fixed mindset approach; cramming for exams at the last minute and retaining information just long enough to pass tests without understanding the material. Despite her best efforts, she was barely passing her courses.

At the end of each semester, Mala took a few days off work to prepare for final exams. She consistently had a low course grade going into her nursing course finals and needed to achieve a certain grade to pass her courses.

By the end of the program, Mala's NCLEX readiness scores were below passing. She continued to work while studying for NCLEX, as bills still had to be paid. Just like when she was in school, Mala resorted to a fixed mindset in her NCLEX preparation. Because she hadn't developed her critical thinking skills during nursing school, she struggled to understand content she needed to learn. She reviewed questions and rationales without learning or understanding question content. After taking hundreds of practice questions, she took NCLEX and failed.

The fallout from this first NCLEX failure was significant. When Mala graduated, she was hired for an RN position in the ED where she had worked as a patient care aide (PCA). Upon graduation, she was promoted to a Nurse Extern position with a moderate pay raise. She would move to her RN position, with an even larger pay raise, when she passed NCLEX. Her failure meant she had to give up her Nurse Extern position and take a pay cut back to her PCA role until she retook and passed NCLEX.

Too embarrassed to seek help from her former instructors, Mala struggled to find effective study strategies on her own. Her financial pressures increased. She had to purchase additional NCLEX preparation materials and pay to retake the exam, all while her student loan repayment began. Without the brain-based learning and critical thinking skills to apply to her NCLEX preparation, Mala failed NCLEX two more times.

Mala's story highlights the hidden costs of overworking while in nursing school—compromised learning, physical exhaustion, missed opportunities for support, and long-term financial and career setbacks.

Emil finding balance.

Emil knew attending nursing school would be challenging, made greater by his need to be fully responsible for his tuition. During the 2 years before he applied and started nursing school, he saved enough to decrease his work hours to part-time during school. He didn't work in health care; he had a job in a warehouse, but he was able to be flexible with his work hours and the pay was acceptable.

Emil knows that when he has too much free time he procrastinates. Because of that, he knew keeping busy would be a good strategy for his success.

When Emil entered his first term with full-time coursework, he reduced his work hours. Each school term, he arranged work hours around his academic needs. He used a handwritten calendar schedule with time blocking. For Emil, writing out this schedule each week on Sunday helped him organize his study time based on his school requirements for the upcoming week.

Prioritizing sleep and focused study time, Emil developed a routine of reviewing class material daily, even if just for 30 min, and incorporated that into his schedule. For his learning, he used brain-based learning techniques, using a growth mindset and applying critical thinking to his learning.

(continued)

When faced with challenging weeks—like when he had multiple exams in one week—Emil planned ahead. He did meal prep, asked for schedule adjustments at work, and communicated with his instructors when he anticipated issues.

Emil wasn't a straight A student. He had to invest in his learning to be successful. There were times he felt overwhelmed or behind. However, he had built a support network of classmates and instructors and wasn't afraid to ask for help. This openness allowed him to address challenges before they became crises.

By the end of the program, Emil had developed strong time management skills along with a deep understanding of nursing concepts. Despite not working in health care while in nursing school, he was able to be successful because he applied his learning to support his ability to think like a nurse.

In his final semester, his NCLEX readiness scores were comfortably above passing. He continued with his part-time work schedule after graduating so that he could commit to NCLEX preparation. He continued creating a weekly schedule each Sunday that included his NCLEX preparation time. Five weeks after graduation, Emil passed NCLEX.

Emil's approach demonstrates how effective time management, open communication, and a focus on balanced learning can lead to success in nursing school, even while working. His story emphasizes the importance of prioritizing education, seeking support, and developing sustainable study habits for long-term success.

Whether you relate more to Mala's struggles, Emil's strategic approach, or your situation is entirely different, effective time management is important for your success.

5.4 Practical Strategies: Managing Your Time

Now that you understand the benefit of time management on your learning, let's review actionable strategies for time management. Use your critical thinking and consider how you can adapt them to fit your unique needs. The goal isn't perfection, but progress. Even small improvements in how you manage your time can lead to significant benefits.

- **Put your schedule in writing**

In whatever format you choose, commit to detailing your schedule by writing it out in an agenda scheduling book, on a calendar, or using an app on your device. Having a set schedule will help you avoid procrastinating and stick to your plans.

- **Schedule study sessions that allow for "chunking" of time**

It is best to schedule study times each day allowing for repetition and integration of your learning. Planning to devote a full 8 h weekend day to study does not support brain-based learning. You will learn better if you review content on an ongoing basis, rather than in long study sessions.

Except for your notes review before and after class, "chunk" study time into intervals. You may already know what your time limit is until you begin to lose focus. This is your "chunk" of time. For many students this is in a range of 20–25 min. Rather than trying to push through that point when you lose focus, set a timer and take a 3–5 min break, between your "chunks" of study time.

- **Schedule study time to review before class**

You will optimize your brain-based learning during class when you begin class focused and ready to enhance your learning of the content you have already reviewed for class. Rushing into class seconds before it begins does not support your learning.

• Schedule study time after each class session

Brain-based learning depends on repetition. Reviewing your class notes for a short period of time right after class will improve integration of your learning.

Keep this in mind when you schedule your classes. If you have the option of creating time breaks between classes, do it. Rushing from one class to the next over a 10 min break will not allow you to optimize your learning.

• Schedule study time without multitasking

Multitasking is a routinely accepted lifestyle behavior but it does not support brain-based learning (May & Elder, 2018; Sana et al., 2013). Schedule study times when you are able to be mindful and focused and without distractions.

Let your friends and family know that during your study time, you won't have your phone. You can create emergency alerts, so if someone does need to get you they can. However, as a routine, turn off devices during your study time. If you are using your computer to study, stop notifications on the computer. You can even install blockers that will prevent you from opening additional windows to reduce your temptation to wander.

If you have difficulty breaking away from your "scrolling," use a tool to monitor phone activity.

Eliminating multitasking will not be easy at first. Just like when you practice mindful relaxation and your brain pulls back to mind chatter, the same is true for your devices. We know they are addictive. When you first go without your phone, or disconnect text and phone alerts from your watch, you will be distracted thinking about what you are missing. You literally are withdrawing from your device. Don't let this stop you from making the change, but recognize why it is happening so you can push through the initial withdrawal.

• Schedule time off

Schedule time off from studying. Time off is important for your overall well-being and will enhance your brain-based learning. If the demands of your schoolwork, job, family, and/or other responsibilities prohibit a day of rest, strive to lighten your load at least 1 day a week.

• Prioritize sleep

You are very busy, and it's tempting to add to your schedule in ways that decrease your sleep time. Remember that getting 6–8 h of sleep each night supports brain-based learning and is essential for your success. When you sleep, the content you learned during the day is processed and consolidated to long-term memory. When you lose a night of sleep, you don't regain that learning during a sleep cycle the following day (McCoy & Strecker, 2011; Poe et al., 2010).

No matter what time scheduling format you use, remember that outlining time for sleep is as important as the time you have for going to class, clinical, and studying.

• Leverage technology

Numerous apps and online tools can enhance your time management. Digital calendars like Google Calendar or Apple Calendar can help you visualize your schedule, set reminders, and share your availability with study groups or clinical supervisors.

While these tools can be incredibly helpful, remember that they're meant to support, not replace, your critical thinking in relation to your time management. Use tools that align with your needs and be sure they are truly enhancing your productivity.

• Reduce time wasting activities

For most everyone, electronic scroll is a common and pervasive time wasting activity. This topic comes up in other chapters because scroll impacts sleep (Chap. 6) stress (Chap. 7) and anxiety (Chap. 8). There are various apps you can use to monitor your online activity, to lock down online resources, even to set a timer for online lock down. Use your critical thinking to decipher what you will need to set limits on activities that go beyond useful downtime.

Keeping these practical strategies in mind as you consider ways to make your time management more effective will contribute to your success.

5.5   Conclusion

Effective time management isn't about cramming more into each day. It's about making smart choices that support your learning, well-being, and success. The skills you develop now will help you balance the demands of nursing school and your life responsibilities.

Improving your time management skills will set you up for success in nursing school, on NCLEX, and in your nursing career. By managing your time well, you're creating space for the critical thinking, brain-based learning, and growth mindset strategies reviewed in Part I. Be patient with yourself as you work to balance your time management. Every small improvement in how you manage your time is a step toward becoming the awesome nurse you're meant to be. Keep at it!

In the next chapter we will review lifestyle factors that you can consider to make your learning easier and more efficient.

Chapter 5 Synthesis Learning Activity: Your Personalized Time Management Plan
The purpose of this learning activity is to create a personalized time management plan that addresses your specific challenges and incorporates strategies you've learned in this chapter. This plan will serve as a practical tool to help you navigate the demands of nursing school.

---

1. Reflect on your current time management practices.
   (a) List your top three time management challenges. These could be issues like procrastination, difficulty balancing work and school, or struggling to find time for self-care.
   (b) Outline a plan to address each of the three challenges.
2. Design a schedule for an upcoming school week that incorporates your chosen strategies. Use Time Blocking or Task Blocking or a format that works best for you.

By completing this activity, you'll have a customized time management plan that addresses your specific needs and challenges as a nursing student. This plan will serve as a practical guide to help you implement the strategies you've learned and make the most of your time in nursing school.

References

May, K. E., & Elder, A. D. (2018). Efficient, helpful, or distracting? A literature review of media multitasking in relation to academic performance. *International Journal of Educational Technology in Higher Education, 15*(1), 1–17.

McCoy, J. G., & Strecker, R. E. (2011). The cognitive cost of sleep lost. *Neurobiology of Learning and Memory, 96*(4), 564–582. https://doi.org/10.1016/j.nlm.2011.07.004

NCSBN. (2024). *NCLEX pass rates*. Retrieved November 4, 2024, from https://www.ncsbn.org/exams/exam-statistics-and-publications/nclex-pass-rates.page

Poe, G. R., Walsh, C. M., & Bjorness, T. E. (2010). Cognitive neuroscience of sleep. *Progress in Brain Research, 185*, 1–19. https://doi.org/10.1016/B978-0-444-53702-7.00001-4

Sana, F., Weston, T., & Cepeda, N. J. (2013). Laptop multitasking hinders classroom learning for both users and nearby peers. *Computers & Education, 62*, 24–31. https://doi.org/10.1016/j.compedu.2012.10.003

Manage Your Lifestyle 6

To keep the body in good health is a duty... otherwise we shall not be able to keep our mind strong and clear.

—*Buddha*

6.1 Introduction

As you progress through your nursing education, you're not just learning medical knowledge and clinical skills—you're also developing the habits and mindset of a nurse. Managing your lifestyle is an important part of this journey. In this chapter we will review daily habits and lifestyle choices that can either support or hinder your learning. These are topics you are familiar with but in this chapter the content is presented to explain "why" and "how" these lifestyle factors support your ability to think critically, use brain-based learning, and adopt a growth mindset. The habits you form now will contribute to your well-being and support your resilience and success in both nursing school and nursing practice.

▶ **By the end of this chapter you will be able to:**
1. Describe the impact of sleep on cognitive function and apply strategies to optimize sleep.
2. Develop a nutrition plan that supports brain health and academic performance.
3. Integrate regular physical activity to improve cognitive function.
4. Implement effective study habits that align with brain-based learning principles.
5. Apply critical thinking skills to assess and modify lifestyle choices for optimal academic and professional success.

6.2 Nursing School Lifestyle

Four key lifestyle factors that are vital for your nursing school success are sleep, nutrition, physical activity, and student behaviors. While each of these elements is important on its own, they work together to help you do your best learning and critical thinking. By understanding and putting into practice good habits in these areas, you'll be better prepared to handle the challenges of nursing school. You'll also develop a healthy lifestyle that will serve you well in your future nursing career. Let's begin our exploration with one of the most basic yet often overlooked aspects of student life: sleep.

© The Author(s), under exclusive license to Springer Nature Switzerland AG 2025
C. Thompson, *Nursing School, NCLEX and Career Transition Success*,
https://doi.org/10.1007/978-3-031-85538-2_6

6.2.1 Sleep

It is essential to make adequate sleep a priority. How much sleep is "adequate"? **Six** to **eight** hours of uninterrupted sleep per night, every night, is the amount recommended by the American Academy of Sleep Medicine (n.d.).

During sleep, your brain processes all that you have learned and experienced in a day. In this section we will break down these stages to understand why 6–8 h of uninterrupted sleep is essential for your learning and overall well-being.

Before we dive into the science of sleep and how it connects to your learning, let's take a look at your current sleep habits. Complete the following Sleep Self-Assessment 6.1 to get a clearer picture of your sleep patterns and habits.

Self-Assessment 6.1: Sleep

You may have a good sleep pattern in which you do get 6–8 uninterrupted hours every night, or you may laugh at that number because you are not able to do that. Taking time to review and reflect on your current sleep behaviors is our starting point for your learning about sleep. You may have an electronic app like a smartwatch that tracks your sleep. If so, use the sleep record of your app for this self-assessment.

Sleep Record

Record your sleep patterns in the last 4 days (if it was a typical activity) on Table 6.1.

For each statement in Table 6.2, check Yes or No.

If you answered "Yes" to most of these questions:

Congratulations! You're on the right track with your sleep habits. Your good sleep routine is supporting your brain-based learning and overall health.

If you answered "No" to many of these questions:

Don't worry—you're not alone. Many nursing students struggle with maintaining

Table 6.1 Sleep record self-assessment

Day	Time to bed	Time awake during the night	Time awake for the day	Total hours of sleep
1				
2				
3				
4				

Table 6.2 Sleep habits self-assessment

My sleep behaviors	Yes	No
In a normal week, I get 6–8 h of uninterrupted sleep per night		
I follow a regular bedtime routine		
I maintain a consistent sleep–wake schedule		
I limit caffeine when it disrupts my sleep		
I limit alcohol		
I avoid screen time for at least 1 h before I go to sleep		
I avoid napping late in the day		
I keep my sleeping area free of clutter		
I love my fur baby (babies) but don't allow them in the bed during the night		
My mattresses and pillows allow for comfortable sleep		
My sleep environment is not impacted by disrupting noises		
I maintain my bedroom at a comfortable temperature for sleep		

healthy sleep habits. The good news is that sleep is a skill you can improve. Implementing even small changes can make a difference in your learning and overall well-being.

Regardless of how you scored, remember that understanding the importance of sleep is the first step toward improvement. Let's now look at why sleep is so crucial for your learning and how you can optimize your sleep habits.

6.2.1.1 Physiology of Sleep

Understanding why good quality sleep is so important for your best academic performance (Curcio et al., 2006) will help you apply your critical thinking when you consider ways to improve your sleep.

During sleep your brain processes all that you have learned and experienced in a day. You've likely already learned in a previous course about the Stages of Sleep. Let's break them down to understand why uninterrupted sleep is essential for brain-based learning.

Non-Rapid Eye Movement (NREM) is the first phase of sleep. During NREM, your body is preparing to enter deep sleep and your brain begins to organize and filter information gathered throughout the day. This leads to a deep phase of NREM sleep where facts and information are consolidated. Also, during NREM sleep, the hippocampus replays the day's experiences to the neocortex, where long-term memories are stored. This replay helps integrate new information with existing knowledge, strengthening memory retention.

During Rapid Eye Movement (REM) sleep, your brain is highly active. In this sleep phase your brain is consolidating procedural memory (how to perform tasks) and emotional memories. Dreams occur in this phase, which is believed to help in processing emotional experiences and integrating new information with existing knowledge.

NREM and REM stages repeat several times throughout the night. Each repeated cycle supports specific aspects of memory processing. Sleep interruptions prevent the brain from completing these cycles and as a result, memories cannot be fully consolidated.

Additionally, NREM and REM sleep promote synaptic plasticity, which is fundamental for learning and memory. In Chap. 2 you learned about the role of neurons and neurotransmitters for relaying information across the synapse to support brain-based learning. This process of synaptic homeostasis strengthens important connections and prunes away less important ones, optimizing the neural network for better memory storage (Poe et al., 2010).

6.2.2 📝 Practical Strategies: Managing Your Sleep

Now that you understand how crucial consistent uninterrupted sleep is for your learning and success, let's review some strategies for improving sleep.

- **Establish a consistent sleep schedule**

  Going to bed and waking up at the same time every day, even on weekends, helps regulate your body's natural sleep–wake cycle. You can't "catch up" on lost sleep, as the interruptions in your regular cycle will not recreate the REM and NREM cycles.

  Consistency reinforces your body's sleep–wake cycle that aligns with your natural circadian rhythms. This helps optimize the timing of different sleep stages, enhancing the memory consolidation and cognitive function that supports your learning.

- **Create a wind down routine before sleep**

  A consistent pre-sleep routine sends information to your brain that it's time to relax. This promotes the release of sleep-inducing hormones like melatonin.

- **Use your bed for the two S's—sleep and sex**

  Don't add a third S—study—to activities you do in bed. Using your bed primarily for sleep creates a strong mental association between your bed and sleep. This will help your brain transition into sleep mode more quickly when you lie down.

- **Avoid screens before bedtime and in bed**

  The blue light emitted from electronic devices can interfere with the production of melatonin and lead to dysregulated sleep. Even though you may be in the habit of watching TV or another electronic device to fall asleep, the activation makes it more difficult for your brain to initiate sleep and reach deep sleep cycles (Randjelović et al., 2023; Yaman Aktaş et al., 2022).

  If your schedule is such that your only choice is to study late at night, utilize filters that limit blue light or invest in a pair of blue light lenses to minimize sleep disruption.

- **When possible, maintain a cool bedroom temperature**

A cooler room temperature helps lower your core body temperature, which is necessary for initiating and maintaining sleep. This promotes deeper, more restorative sleep stages that are required for memory consolidation.

Not everyone has optimal housing. If you have the option to control your bedroom temperature, keep it cool. If you don't, work to address other strategies to improve your sleep.

- **Align sleep with natural sleep–wake cycles**

Your body's circadian rhythm is strongly influenced by light exposure. It is best to wake up to natural sunlight. This helps reset your circadian rhythm daily, improving daytime alertness and nighttime sleep quality. Sleep in darkness to promote melatonin production, which signals your brain it's time for restorative sleep.

If your sleep–wake cycles can't align with natural daylight/night cycles (e.g., if you work night shifts), use a sleep mask to simulate darkness during your sleep hours and consider using a light lighting that mimics natural sunlight.

Aligning your sleep patterns with natural light cycles, or simulating them when necessary, supports your brain's innate rhythms and as a result, optimal learning, memory consolidation, and overall cognitive performance in your nursing studies (Irish et al., 2015).

- **Limit caffeine, alcohol, and other stimulant drugs**

Caffeine is a stimulant that you metabolize based on your genetics. As you know some people can have a cup of cappuccino right before bed and feel it has not affected their sleep, while others can't have a decaf coffee after 10 AM. Depending on how you metabolize it, caffeine can stay in your system for up to 8 h and interfere with your ability to fall asleep or stay in deep sleep (Irish et al., 2015). Know and respect how caffeine impacts your sleep.

Unlike caffeine, alcohol impacts everyone consistently. It makes you feel sleepy initially but then disrupts REM sleep and leads to more frequent wake-ups during the night.

If you take medication for an attention disorder you already know how the medication keeps your brain alert. Make good choices about the timing of stimulant medications so that your sleep is not affected.

There are a variety of other drugs and medications that interfere with sleep. Avoid using them. Beyond the impact on your sleep, you are taking significant risks for reaching your goal of becoming a nurse. An arrest or other drug-related crime on your record can have far-reaching consequences for your ability to get clearance for clinical while in school or to get approved for licensure after you graduate.

- **Manage stress and anxiety**

If you struggle with stress and anxiety, you know these emotions make sleep more difficult. These emotions activate your sympathetic nervous system, making it difficult to fall asleep and reducing sleep quality (Sanford et al., 2015; Zhang et al., 2018). Strategies for reducing stress, managing unavoidable stress, and for addressing anxiety as it relates to nursing school and test anxiety are reviewed in Chaps. 7 and 8.

- **Practice relaxation techniques**

Particularly helpful if you struggle with stress or anxiety, relaxation techniques activate the parasympathetic nervous system, countering stress responses and preparing your brain and body for restful sleep. More detailed information about managing stress is reviewed in Chap. 7 and in Chap. 8.

- **Exercise regularly**

The next section of this chapter reviews more about the benefits of physical activity for your learning. In relation to sleep; regular exercise promotes better sleep quality and duration. However, exercising too close to bedtime can be

6.2 Nursing School Lifestyle

stimulating, so the timing of your physical activity is important for optimal sleep.

- **Keep pets out of the bed; if they disrupt sleep, out of the bedroom**

We love our furry friends, and they can provide comfort and alleviate anxiety; however, pets can disrupt sleep cycles with their movements or noises that interrupt sleep, interfering with your ability to get the best learning support that comes with good quality, uninterrupted sleep.

When you are making choices to improve your sleep use your critical thinking skills to analyze your habits and identify areas where you can make improvements. Make addressing sleep a priority for brain-based learning. Pause and Reflect 6.1 will help you develop a plan for improving your sleep.

Pause and Reflect 6.1: Better Sleep for Better Learning

Now that you have a better understanding of the importance of sleep as it relates to your nursing school success, reflect on your self-assessment and lifestyle adjustments you can make if you determine that your sleep is less than optimal.

1. Review your sleep record and self-assessment (Self-Assessment 6.1). How might your current sleep patterns be impacting your ability to learn and retain information in your nursing studies?
2. Now that you understand the importance of NREM and REM sleep cycles for memory consolidation and cognitive function, which aspects of your sleep habits might be hindering these processes?
3. Identify sleep recommendations that you believe would have the most significant impact on optimizing your learning. What specific steps can you take to implement change for each recommendation?

6.2.3 Nutrition

As a nursing student you learn about the importance of nutrition in supporting health. In addition to supporting overall physical health and in many cases, managing health conditions, your nutrition also plays a role in brain function that supports learning. This section covers the basics of nutrition related to optimizing brain-based learning. Individual needs vary, and these guidelines should be adapted to your personal health requirements, cultural background, and economic circumstances. Dietary choices are deeply personal and influenced by cultural, religious, and ethical considerations.

Nutrition Essentials to Support Brain Function

The foods listed here are examples of nutrient-rich options that are specific to brain function but this is not an exhaustive list. Many cultures have traditional foods that offer similar benefits. The goal of this section is to provide you with knowledge to make choices about your diet, considering foods that support your ability to learn.

- **Omega-3 Fatty Acids**

Omega-3 fatty acids are essential for brain health. They are associated with increased learning, memory, cognitive well-being, and improved blood flow in the brain. These fatty acids help build cell membranes in the brain and reduce inflammation, which is linked to neurodegenerative diseases (Dyall, 2015; Gómez-Pinilla, 2008).

Sources in salmon, walnuts, flaxseeds, chia seeds, and soybeans.

- **Antioxidants**

Antioxidants help protect brain cells from oxidative stress, which can damage cells and contribute to aging and neurodegenerative diseases. They also promote neurogenesis (the growth of new neurons) and improve synaptic plasticity, which is essential for learning and memory (Poulose et al., 2017).

Sources include: Dark vegetables (broccoli, spinach, carrots, sweet potatoes); dark fruits (fresh or dried blueberries, blackberries, cherries, raspberries, cranberries); beans (red kidney beans, black beans, pinto beans); spices (turmeric, cinnamon, oregano, cumin, curry powder, peppermint); and beverages (tea or coffee in moderation, apple juice, grapefruit juice).

- **Whole Grains**

Whole grains provide a steady supply of glucose, the brain's primary energy source. They are also rich in fiber, which helps regulate blood sugar levels and prevent energy crashes that affect cognitive function.

Sources include brown rice, whole wheat bread, and oatmeal.

- **Cholines**

Choline is a vital nutrient for brain health. It is a precursor to acetylcholine, a neurotransmitter involved in many functions, including memory and muscle control. Adequate choline intake supports cognitive function, brain development, and may protect against cognitive decline (Blusztajn et al., 2017).

Sources include eggs, beef liver, chicken, fish, peanuts, and cruciferous vegetables (Brussels sprouts, broccoli), and peas.

And last but not least:

- **Hydration**

Adequate hydration is essential for optimal brain function. Dehydration can impair short-term memory, attention, and long-term memory recall. Water (not sugary drinks) is critical for maintaining the balance of bodily fluids and for the efficient functioning of neurotransmitter systems in the brain (Masento et al., 2014).

6.3 📋 Practical Strategies: Managing Your Nutrition

Following the nutrition recommendations described when you are in nursing school can be tricky. Limited time, tight budgets, and limited access to these food options can make implementing a healthy diet lifestyle challenging. However, with some critical thinking you can decide how to act on making changes that are realistic.

- **Consider budget-friendly brain foods**

Eating healthy doesn't mean you have to break the bank. If you are looking to add essential omega-e fatty acids, canned tuna or sardines are more affordable than salmon.

In season fruits and vegetables are less costly than out of season, but frozen fruits and vegetables are often cheaper than fresh and retain their nutritional value.

Looking for protein and choline? Eggs can be a cost-effective source of both. And beans and lentils offer affordable protein and fiber alternatives to meat.

- **Adopt time-saving strategies**

Who has extra time in nursing school? However, consider preparing meals in bulk when you have term or semester breaks. Freeze in single use portions for a healthy meal on busy days.

Keep healthy snacks at the ready to reduce your dependence on processed foods for snacking. Nutrient-dense snacks like nuts, Greek yogurt, homemade trail mix, a banana, or cut vegetables offer whole food healthy options on the go.

Plan ahead with packed meals and healthy snacks for long class or clinical days. Rushing for quick snacks is the place where you are most likely to find less healthy options.

- **Consider easy swaps**

Replace soda with water or unsweetened tea. This simple change can significantly reduce your sugar intake, reduce costs and improve hydration.

Choose whole grains instead of white breads for more sustained energy.

- **Make the most of campus dining options**

If you have access to campus dining, consider making healthy choices there.

6.4 Practical Strategies: Physical Activity

- Look for salad bars and customize with brain-boosting ingredients like leafy greens, nuts, and lean proteins.
- Choose grilled options over fried foods when possible.
- Avoid the soda machines and dessert bars.

When you are making choices to improve your eating habits to support your learning, remember, perfection isn't the goal. Small, consistent changes can make a big difference. Use your critical thinking skills to analyze your current eating habits and identify areas where you can make improvements. Every healthy choice, no matter how small, is a step toward optimizing your brain function and supporting your success in nursing school. And speaking of steps…

6.3.1 Physical Activity

What you are learning in this book is the relationship between behaviors and your nursing school success, so here we will look at the link between physical activity and brain-based learning. You already know that physical activity is important. Nurses include this in health promotion and disease prevention patient education for a number of health conditions.

You may be surprised to learn that physical activity is strongly correlated to brain function (Cotman et al., 2007). The multiple benefits of physical activity and links to learning are shown in Table 6.3.

You see that being physically active not only benefits your physical health, but also boosts your brain function in a number of different ways.

Embracing changes in your physical activity is an individualized decision and impacted by many factors; some of which you may not be able to control. You may already have a routine of physical activity that is a part of your regular lifestyle habits, or on the other hand, you may have limitations that are difficult to control. Understanding the benefits of physical activity for improving your learning, again, the "why" and "how," may serve as a motivator for you to make changes to move around more.

Table 6.3 Physical activity and learning

Benefit of physical activity	How it supports brain function
Enhanced blood flow and oxygen delivery	Increases heart rate and blood flow Improves delivery of oxygen and nutrients to the brain Enhances concentration, memory, and mental clarity
Neurogenesis and synaptic plasticity	Promotes creation of new neurons, especially in the hippocampus Enhances brain's ability to form new synaptic connections Fundamental for memory formation and learning
Mood regulation and stress reduction	Triggers release of endorphins Reduces stress, anxiety, and depression Creates a more conducive environment for learning
Improved sleep quality	Helps regulate sleep patterns Supports memory consolidation and cognitive processes
Enhanced executive function	Improves planning, problem-solving, and multitasking Leads to better organizational skills and study habits Helps with time management and task prioritization
Increased brain-derived neurotrophic factor (BDNF)	Supports survival, growth, and differentiation of neurons Enhances learning capabilities Helps protect against cognitive decline

6.4 📝 Practical Strategies: Physical Activity

If you are not in the routine of getting regular physical activity, you don't have to commit hours of your time to get these amazing benefits to support your learning. You can take simple steps if you're starting from scratch.

- **Add steps whenever possible**

When you make an intention to add more steps in your daily activity (this isn't something you will have to be intentional about when you begin your nursing career and practice clinical nursing at the bedside!) you can discover hidden opportunities to move. If you drive to campus, allow yourself an extra 10 min, park farther away to walk further. When you drive for errands, park farther from entrances to add more steps. When it is feasible and safe, walk or bike instead of driving. Take the stairs instead of the elevator. Replace 10 min of morning scroll through social media with a 10 min walk. Once you apply your critical thinking to the question "how can I add more steps?" you will find many answers.

- **Use active study techniques**

You can't get away from having to spend time sitting; on average, you should be spending about 3 h of study time for every 1 h of class time. That is a lot of sitting! Consider ways to move while you study. Do you have an area where you can stand instead of sitting? Take a walk while you listen to recorded lectures. Recall the brain-based learning principle of "chunking" your study time? When you take your break after 20 min, take a short walk, do jumping jacks or squats.

- **Utilize campus resources**

Many schools have campus gyms and exercise facilities that are available to students. This is a rare opportunity for you to have free access to this type of resource. Typically, these facilities are open early in the morning and late into the evening and offer a variety of options for physical activity.

- **Combine socializing with activity**

Instead of meeting friends for coffee, suggest a walk or active outing. This allows you to maintain social connections while increasing your physical activity.

- **Schedule physical activity**

Consider including physical activity in your time management schedule. If you tend to procrastinate about making time for physical activity, treating it as an important appointment increases the likelihood you'll follow through.

- **Engage in activities you enjoy**

Physical activity takes many forms. You don't have to start running, take long walks, or go to a class at the gym. Incorporate activities you enjoy that include movement, such as gardening, or dancing. When exercise is fun, you're more likely to stick with it.

If you do need to boost your physical activity, as you consider ways to do that, keep in mind the goal isn't to overhaul your life but to make sustainable changes that support your brain health and learning capacity.

Consider your daily schedule, your living situation, and your personal preferences. Which of these strategies could you realistically implement? How might you modify them to fit your unique circumstances? Perhaps you could start with just one or two changes and gradually add more as they become a habit.

By approaching physical activity with the same critical thinking you apply to your nursing studies, you can develop a plan that enhances your cognitive function and supports your academic success. Every bit of movement counts toward supporting your brain health and learning potential.

Now that you see the benefits of sleep, nutrition, and physical activity in supporting your lifestyle for nursing school success, let's review one last factor, your student behaviors.

6.4.1 Student Behavior

In Part I "Foundation for Thinking and Learning in Nursing School" you learned about the importance of critical thinking and using brain-based learning strategies and a growth mindset to support your success. Just as your choices about sleep, nutrition, and physical activity can significantly impact your cognitive function and learning capacity, the way you approach your studies and engage with your education is equally important. You can support your learning by adopting habits of high performing students.

High-performing nursing students integrate these foundational concepts into their daily academic routines. They:

- Apply critical thinking not just to course content, but to their own learning process.
- Structure their study habits around brain-based learning principles rather than falling back on less effective memorization techniques.
- Maintain a growth mindset even when faced with challenging content or disappointing grades.
- View each class, clinical, and simulation as an opportunity for learning rather than just tasks to complete.

Success in nursing school requires more than just showing up to class or clinical. The student behaviors you adopt will contribute to or hinder your academic success.

6.5 Practical Strategies: Student Behaviors

These behaviors and habits of high performing students don't just apply when you are in nursing school. These are habits and behaviors that, when you carry them into your professional role as a nurse, will support your success.

- **Attend class and clinical**

Your nursing program may have an attendance policy but your growth mindset, rather than a program requirement, should be your incentive to not miss class or clinical. Class and clinical contribute to your learning by adding opportunity for interleaving, repetition, and reflection, all aspects of brain-based learning.

- **Stay fully engaged in your class learning**

Attending class but tuning out the learning is the same as not going at all. Stay engaged with your learning by adopting the following behaviors as your routine:

(a) Turn off your devices to avoid distractions. Only use your devices when you are looking up something to enhance your learning.

(b) Prepare for class even when pre-reading is not required. Brain-based learning is supported by interleaving and repetition. You may not understand the reading before class, but exposing yourself to the content will support your integration when you see and hear it again in class.

(c) Participate in in-class learning activities. If you are in a learning activity group that is not staying on task, take a leadership role and put the learning back on task. If you or your group are off task because you don't understand the project, ask the instructor for help.

(d) Choose your seat in the classroom with intention. If you are easily distracted, don't sit by the door or window. If sitting in the front helps you stay engaged, choose a front row seat.

(e) If you're an introvert, fight the urge to resist asking questions in class. Clarifying information as you are learning supports interleaving.

Your commitment to staying engaged in class will enhance your learning.

- **Stay fully engaged in your clinical learning**

Clinical time is as valuable as classroom time but offers more variability in learning opportunities. Approach your clinical with a growth mindset, applying critical thinking to your learning. Even when there's a shortage of clinical preceptors or periods of unsupervised downtime, it's crucial to remain focused on learning rather than studying for other exams or engaging in nonclinical activities.

Below are suggestions for clinical activities with critical thinking to support your learning:

(a) Review your client's medication list.

- Why is each medication on the list prescribed for this client?
- What potential drug interactions should the nurse be alert for?

(b) Review your client's laboratory and imaging:
- Why was this test ordered?
- How do the test findings support or contraindicate the medical conditions?

(c) Consider preventative aspects of your client's care:
- Could this hospitalization (or illness) have been prevented?
- What lifestyle factors on the part of the client might have contributed to medical conditions client is experiencing?

(d) Consider expected outcomes of your client's care:
- What criteria will the client need to meet to be ready for discharge?
- What is the typical trajectory for a client with this condition?

(e) Practice giving a change of shift report to a fellow student.
- What are the care priorities?
- What lab values and diagnostic test results will indicate the client is making progress?
- What are the most crucial teaching points for the nurse to address?

(f) Observe and analyze interprofessional interactions:
- How do different health care professionals communicate and collaborate?
- What roles do various team members play in client care?

(g) Seek opportunities to perform or assist with procedures:
- Ask your preceptor or other staff if you can observe or assist with procedures.
- Practice explaining procedures to clients (with supervision).

Making the most of your clinical time will support your learning and your ability to apply critical thinking to your clinical decision making and clinical judgment.

- **Connect with your instructors**

Even if you are an introvert, make an effort to engage with your nursing instructors. Many nursing students consider their instructors to be "unapproachable." Your nursing instructors are nurses. They are caring individuals who have a passion for teaching nursing.

Keep in mind that your instructor's classroom presence may not reflect their true approachability. Teaching a class requires a great deal of focus and concentration. Your instructors are managing the classroom, delivering content effectively, observing student comprehension, and keeping an eye on the clock. This intense focus may make them appear less approachable than they really are. You may find when you meet your instructor one-on-one during an office hour appointment they are more relaxed and personable than they appeared to be in the classroom.

Don't hesitate to visit during office hours or make appointments to discuss your questions or concerns. Their dedication to your success often becomes more apparent in one-on-one interactions.

- **Focus on your learning, not on your grades**

If you are concerned about a grade you earned on an assignment, don't approach your instructor about it when you are angry or upset. First, review the assignment and the grading rubric. You may have worked hard but gone off target on the assignment expectations. Ask your instructor to help you understand how you could have done better.

Likewise, if you are concerned about an exam grade, don't take a confrontational approach when you meet with your instructor. Your instructor has more expertise with the exam topics than you. Ask your instructor to help you understand the content and application of the content to the questions you missed.

- **Join and actively participate in nursing student groups**

Your school of nursing should have a student nurse organization where you can engage with and learn from fellow students. This will give you valuable peer support as well as connection to

6.5 Practical Strategies: Student Behaviors

students in higher level courses who can provide suggestions to help you navigate your learning.

- **Develop strong study habits**

Include study times in your schedule. Regular study times will help reinforce learning and ensure you are frequently reviewing material, which enhances brain-based learning.

Optimize your study time by doing the following:

(a) Schedule a 30 min study time after each class session. This immediate review of content supports the repetition that is essential for brain-based learning.
(b) Avoid distractions. Plan your study time when you know you can be totally focused on studying.
(c) Don't multitask during your study time.
(d) Create a dedicated study space. Having a specific area for studying can help your brain associate that space with focus and learning.
(e) Review material regularly. Don't wait until just before exams.

- **Use active learning study strategies**

Use active learning techniques when you are studying. Techniques such as summarizing, using flashcards, questioning, study group discussion and teaching others can reinforce your understanding and retention of information.

- **Seek feedback and use it constructively**

Regularly ask your instructors for feedback and receive it with a growth mindset. Reflect on the feedback and identify areas for improvement. Create a plan to incorporate the feedback into your learning and behaviors.

- **Utilize school resources**

Remain proactive in accessing the resources available to you. Don't wait until you are falling behind in a course. Your school should provide academic support as well as counseling and mental health resources. Know when you need help and seek it out.

- **Practice self-care**

What are you supposed to do if you're on a plane that's in trouble and the oxygen masks come down? You put your own mask on before helping others. Keep this in mind for your self-care. Give yourself the oxygen first. Maintain a healthy work–life balance. Use whatever mindfulness and stress relief strategies work to keep you in balance.

- **Redirect focus in content that is not interesting to you**

You won't love every class session, clinical experience, or course in your nursing school. Your attitude impacts learning. When you feel a negative attitude setting in, be aware of it and use your critical thinking skills to reset from the negative attitude to a growth mindset.

- **Build professional relationships**

Practice taking on a professional demeanor while you are still in school. Network with your instructors and with clinicians. Find a mentor to role model. If given the opportunity, attend a professional conference.

By incorporating these additional behaviors, you can further enhance your learning experience and set yourself up for success in nursing school and beyond.

Pause and Reflect 6.2 will give you an opportunity to think back on one of your best learning experiences and consider how your student behaviors contributed to success.

Pause and Reflect 6.2: Your Best Learning Experience

Think back to a course or learning experience where you excelled and genuinely enjoyed the learning process. This could be from nursing school or any previous educational experience.

Reflect on the following questions:

1. What made this learning experience stand out for you? Was it the subject matter, the

teaching style, your personal approach, or a combination of factors?

2. How engaged were you in this course? Consider your attendance, participation in class discussions, and preparation for each session.

3. What study habits did you employ? Did you use any specific strategies for note-taking, reviewing material, or preparing for exams?

4. What behaviors or attitudes contributed to your success?

By reflecting on a past success, you can identify the behaviors and attitudes that contributed to your achievement. Use these insights to reinforce positive habits in your nursing education and to approach challenging courses with strategies you know have worked for you in the past. Replicating the elements of success from your previous experiences will support your current and future success.

6.6 Conclusion

This chapter explored four important lifestyle factors that impact your ability to learn, think critically, and succeed in nursing school. Optimizing sleep, nourishing your brain with the right foods, incorporating physical activity, and adopting effective student behaviors each have equal parts in contributing to your success. These lifestyle choices are not just about getting through nursing school, they are about developing healthy habits and behaviors that will serve you in your nursing career.

In the next chapter we will take a look at stress and consider ways for you to manage the stress that is so much a part of your life as a nursing student. Just like with the other topics in the book, you'll learn about "why" and "how" stress impacts you and ways you can reduce your stress.

Table 6.4 Lifestyle synthesis learning activity table

Category	Behavior to adjust	Barriers to change	Solutions
Sleep			
Nutrition			
Physical activity			
Study habits			
Engagement with learning			
Attitude			

Chapter 6 Synthesis Learning Activity: Lifestyle Lab—Optimal Learning

The purpose of this learning activity is to apply critical thinking to identify lifestyle factors reviewed in the chapter that serve you well, and areas where you could make changes to support your success.

Reflect on your current lifestyle habits and how they align with the principles of brain-based learning discussed in this chapter. Complete Table 6.4 to identify behaviors you want to adjust, potential barriers to making that change, and practical solutions to overcome those barriers.

References

American Academy of Sleep Medicine. (n.d.). *Sleep deprivation.* https://aasm.org/resources/factsheets/sleepdeprivation.pdf

Blusztajn, J. K., Slack, B. E., & Mellott, T. J. (2017). Neuroprotective actions of dietary choline. *Nutrients, 9*(8), 815. https://doi.org/10.3390/nu9080815

Cotman, C. W., Berchtold, N. C., & Christie, L. A. (2007). Exercise builds brain health: Key roles of growth factor cascades and inflammation. *Trends in Neurosciences, 30*(9), 464–472.

Curcio, G., Ferrara, M., & De Gennaro, L. (2006). Sleep loss, learning capacity and academic performance. *Sleep Medicine Reviews, 10*(5), 323–337. https://doi.org/10.1016/j.smrv.2005.11.001

Dyall, S. C. (2015). Long-chain omega-3 fatty acids and the brain: A review of the independent and shared effects of EPA, DPA and DHA. *Frontiers in Aging Neuroscience, 7*, 52. https://doi.org/10.3389/fnagi.2015.00052

References

Gómez-Pinilla, F. (2008). Brain foods: The effects of nutrients on brain function. *Nature Reviews Neuroscience, 9*(7), 568–578. https://doi.org/10.1038/nrn2421

Irish, L. A., Kline, C. E., Gunn, H. E., Buysse, D. J., & Hall, M. H. (2015). The role of sleep hygiene in promoting public health: A review of empirical evidence. *Sleep Medicine Reviews, 22*, 23–36. https://doi.org/10.1016/j.smrv.2014.10.001

Masento, N. A., Golightly, M., Field, D. T., Butler, L. T., & van Reekum, C. M. (2014). Effects of hydration status on cognitive performance and mood. *British Journal of Nutrition, 111*(10), 1841–1852. https://doi.org/10.1017/S0007114513004455

Poe, G. R., Walsh, C. M., & Bjorness, T. E. (2010). Cognitive neuroscience of sleep. *Progress in Brain Research, 185*, 1–19. https://doi.org/10.1016/B978-0-444-53702-7.00001-4

Poulose, S. M., Miller, M. G., Scott, T., & Shukitt-Hale, B. (2017). Nutritional factors affecting adult neurogenesis and cognitive function. *Advances in Nutrition, 8*(6), 804–811. https://doi.org/10.3945/an.117.016261

Randjelović, P., Stojanović, N., Ilić, I., & Vučković, D. (2023). The effect of reducing blue light from smartphone screen on subjective quality of sleep among students. *Chronobiology International, 40*(3), 335–342. https://doi.org/10.1080/07420528.2023.2173606

Sanford, L. D., Suchecki, D., & Meerlo, P. (2015). Stress, arousal, and sleep. In *Sleep, neuronal plasticity and brain function* (pp. 379–410). Springer.

Yaman Aktaş, Y., Karabulut, N., & Arslan, B. (2022). Digital addiction, academic performance, and sleep disturbance among nursing students. *Perspectives in Psychiatric Care, 58*(4), 1537–1545. https://doi.org/10.1111/ppc.12961

Zhang, Y., Peters, A., & Chen, G. (2018). Perceived stress mediates the associations between sleep quality and symptoms of anxiety and depression among college nursing students. *International Journal of Nursing Education Scholarship, 15*(1), 201–220. https://doi.org/10.1515/ijnes-2017-0020

Manage Stress

7

It's not stress that kills us, it is our reaction to it.

—Hans Selye

7.1 Introduction

As a nursing student, you're no stranger to stress. The demanding nature of your program, coupled with personal responsibilities and the pressure to excel, can create a perfect storm of stressors. Effective stress management is not just about surviving nursing school—it's a skill set that will serve you throughout your nursing career. In this chapter, we'll explore the various sources of stress you may encounter, understand how they impact your learning and well-being, and develop strategies to manage them effectively.

▶ **By the end of this chapter you will be able to:**
1. Differentiate between stress and anxiety, and identify common sources of stress for nursing students.
2. Analyze how stress affects brain-based learning and academic performance.
3. Evaluate current stress levels and identify personal stressors using self-assessment tools.
4. Develop a personalized stress management plan incorporating various coping strategies.

5. Apply critical thinking skills and a growth mindset to address and mitigate stress-inducing situations.

7.2 Stress and Anxiety

Effective stress management is essential for your well-being. As a nursing student you have stressors similar to other students in higher education, and stressors that are unique to nursing education. These unique stressors include competition to succeed and progress in the nursing program, clinical experience and expectations, and high stakes testing (Turner & McCarthy, 2017). These stressors are cumulative and can significantly impact ability to focus, learn, and be successful in nursing school (Heinrich & O'Connell, 2024; Uysal & Çalışkan, 2022).

Stress and anxiety are often used interchangeably, and while related, are distinct experiences with different causes and manifestations. Strategies for managing anxiety are reviewed in Chap. 8.

Stress is your body's response to demands or challenges. It can be positive, motivating you to meet deadlines or perform well on exams. When

© The Author(s), under exclusive license to Springer Nature Switzerland AG 2025
C. Thompson, *Nursing School, NCLEX and Career Transition Success*,
https://doi.org/10.1007/978-3-031-85538-2_7

Table 7.1 Characteristics of stress and anxiety

Stress	Anxiety
Body's response to specific demands or challenges	A persistent feeling of worry or fear
Can be positive (eustress) or negative (distress)	More negative than positive
Typically tied to identifiable external factors or events	Often not tied to a specific external trigger and persists in the absence of immediate stressors
Can motivate performance or overwhelm when chronic	May involve anticipation of future threats
May subside when the stressor is removed	Tends to be long-lasting

stress becomes chronic or overwhelming, it can be negative and impact your physical and mental health, as well as your academic performance (Windle & Musselman, 2022). Unlike anxiety, which can persist without a clear external trigger, stress is typically tied to specific events or circumstances (Lazarus, 1984; American Psychological Association, 2022). Understanding this distinction is crucial for developing effective coping strategies. Table 7.1 outlines the characteristics of stress and anxiety.

Certain low levels of stress, known as eustress, can actually enhance performance and motivation. This positive stress can help you stay focused, meet deadlines, and perform well on exams. The key is to manage stress levels so they remain in this productive range, rather than becoming overwhelming.

Differentiating between stress and anxiety can be helpful to reduce the potential to be overwhelmed. Identifying external stressors that impact you and putting strategies in place to manage them improves your ability to learn.

7.3 Common Stressors for Nursing Students

As a nursing student, you have multiple stressors, some you can reduce, others, you can be aware of and manage your response to the stress. Let's review some of the stressors that you are likely to experience in nursing school.

7.3.1 Time and Performance Pressure

Nursing school is busy. In addition to the rigor of nursing school, most nursing students work while they are in school. And there are family obligations and other important activities. In addition, nursing school requires performing at a certain level to get into the program and then performing to stay in the program. These time and performance stressors can become overwhelming stressors.

A factor that compounds these stressors for nursing students is being surrounded by others who are also dealing with the same pressures. As individuals, we are not closed systems. We are open systems and our bodies absorb the energy from those around us.

Think about how you feel when you're out with friends at a fun and happy event; maybe a party or a wedding. Your body feels light and energized when you are sharing joy with your friends. The opposite is true when you are in class or clinical with student peers who are stressed. You can feel their stress, and it can accelerate your own feelings of stress.

The rigorous time demands, combined with your individual and shared stress while you are in nursing school, contribute to time and performance pressure. The stress of these factors can impact your ability to apply brain-based learning, adopt a growth mindset, and use critical thinking when you approach your learning. Identifying these stressors and implementing strategies to mitigate them will improve your ability to succeed. Let's begin with a self-assessment of your time and performance pressure. Complete Self-Assessment 7.1.

Self-Assessment 7.1: Time and Performance Pressure

The purpose of this two-part self-assessment is to evaluate your priorities for how to spend

7.4 Practical Strategies: Managing Time and Performance Pressures

Table 7.2 Weekly activity by % in self-assessment

Day of week	% in class	% Studying	% at work	% Friends	% Family	% Doing nothing	% Other
Monday							
Tuesday							
Wednesday							
Thursday							
Friday							
Saturday							
Sunday							

your time while in nursing school and the impact of performance pressure on your day to day life as a nursing student.

Part 1: Time Pressure

Complete Table 7.2 to see an overview of how you spend your time in a typical nursing school week.

Reflect on the following questions.

1. Do you have work obligations that impact time pressure? If so, to what extent and do you have options you could consider to adjust that?
2. Do you have family obligations that put pressure on your time? If so, what temporary adjustments can you make while you are in nursing school?
3. Are you overcommitted to something else that creates time pressure? If so, what adjustments can you make while you are in nursing school?
4. Is your "doing nothing" column more than it should be? If so, what strategies can you use to manage your procrastination?

Part 2: Performance Pressure

Complete Table 7.3 to begin your performance pressure self-assessment.

1. How does your performance pressure score align with your time pressure assessment?
2. Which aspects of performance in nursing school cause you the most stress?
3. How might your time management affect your performance pressure, and vice versa?

Table 7.3 Performance pressure self-assessment

Statement	1	2	3	4	5
I feel pressured by the academic expectations in nursing school					
I feel pressured about maintaining the GPA required to stay in the program					
I feel pressured to pass each of my nursing courses					
I feel pressured to compete academically with my peers					
I feel pressured about clinical performance evaluations					
I feel pressured when preparing for exams or important assignments					
I feel pressured about meeting deadlines for assignment deadlines					
Total					

Rate your agreement on a scale of 1–5
(1 = Strongly Disagree, 5 = Strongly Agree)
Scoring:
　7–15: Low performance pressure.
　16–25: Moderate performance pressure.
　26–35: High performance pressure

Now that you have taken time to consider your time and performance pressure, let's look at strategies you can consider to address these overlapping pressures while you are in nursing school.

7.4　Practical Strategies: Managing Time and Performance Pressures

1. Evaluate the impact of work

It is important to find a balance that allows you to meet your financial needs without compromising your academic performance. If your self-assessment revealed to you that work pressure interferes with your ability to succeed, review the section in Chap. 5. You may discover there are alternatives to ease your time pressure burdens from work.

2. **Identify commitments that can be temporarily reduced**

Nursing school is a moment in time. It feels overwhelming right now and you may even feel like you can't see the end, but it will end. You won't be confined to these rigorous demands forever. Reevaluate activities you include in your schedule "because you've always done that."

3. **Set realistic goals**

Break down performance goals into small, achievable milestones. Looking at the entire semester workload is overwhelming. Instead, focus on what you will accomplish today, this week, before next week.

4. **Develop strong time management skills**

Create and stick to a study schedule, using tools like planners or digital apps to manage your time efficiently. Break large tasks into smaller, manageable chunks, and allocate specific time slots for different activities. For more detailed strategies on time management, refer back to Chap. 5.

5. **Evaluate "down-time"**

During nursing school "down-time" is important but there can be a fine line between "down-time" and procrastination. If you tend to procrastinate, review Chap. 5 and consider using a time schedule strategy to help you stay on track.

6. **Commit to a growth mindset**

Focusing on your learning over your performance compared to others will decrease your stress. While grades are important, emphasize a deep understanding of material.

7. **Maintain your perspective**

Remember why you chose nursing. Connecting with your passion can help you push through difficult times and keep proper perspective when you don't score as well as you'd like on a course or clinical assignment. Your performance on one assignment or one exam will not define you as a nurse.

8. **Keep track of your overall grades**

Earning a lower than expected grade in one assignment may leave you feeling discouraged but that one assignment may not significantly impact your overall course grade. Keep the broader perspective of your overall course learning and success rather than focusing on one assignment or exam.

9. **Prioritize**

Not everything that feels urgent is truly important. Focus on high-priority items that are both urgent and important, scheduling less critical tasks for later. When you are overwhelmed, it feels less stressful to tackle the easy tasks first, but they may not be the most important. Assess your priorities as deadlines approach and new assignments are added.

10. **Develop effective study strategies**

Quality of study time is more important than quantity. Use active learning techniques that help you improve understanding and retention so you can apply your critical thinking throughout your learning. These include active learning activities that support brain-based learning such as summarizing key points, teaching concepts to peers, or creating concept maps to visualize connections between ideas.

11. **Note your peer influences**

Pay attention to those around you; what stressor are they bringing into your energy? If before class, chatter centers around negative talk like "this class is the worst!" or "I know I'm going to fail the next test," separate yourself. Find a support system of like-minded peers who will be focusing on healthy stress management.

12. **Practice stress-reduction techniques**

You can't activate your sympathetic (stress response) nervous system and your parasympathetic (relaxed state) nervous system at the same time. When you activate your parasympathetic nervous system you move away from your stress response. Deep breathing, meditation, and mindfulness are just a few examples of activities you can use when you feel external pressure.

13. **Don't compare yourself to others**

You may have been a high performer before you came to nursing school and found yourself now earning grades that are lower than you were used to. Nursing school is difficult. Do not let your grades define you or your ability to be a nurse.

14. **Know when to seek help**

With all of the stressors you face, a good management strategy to adopt it to know when to seek help, and to seek it. Resources should be available to you through your nursing school, but there are also many readily available online and in person resources to provide you with the help you need when things feel like they are getting too difficult to manage.

These strategies will support your ability to manage performance pressure in nursing school.

> **Nursing School Application: Time and Performance Pressure: Time Runs Out and Performance Suffers**
>
> This scenario demonstrates how the external factors of time and performance stress impacts a student who does not use strategies to manage the time and performance pressure.

Sam is approaching the final exam for his first nursing course. Throughout the semester, he's maintained his usual routine of attending classes and clinicals but hasn't established a regular study schedule. His strategy of paying attention in class and cramming the night before exams, which served him well in high school and prerequisite courses, is not working in this first nursing course that requires critical thinking and application of learning.

Like many nursing students, Sam's schedule is packed. He works part-time in the campus Admissions office, maintains an active social life, and constantly communicates via text and social media. Despite the increasing complexity of the coursework, Sam has continually postponed in-depth studying, telling himself he'll "catch up later."

As the semester progressed, Sam missed several opportunities to attend office hours, convinced he could manage on his own. Now, with the final exam looming, he's calculated that he needs an 80% to pass the course. The realization hits him: the stakes are higher than ever before.

The evening before the final, Sam settles in for a long study session. As he reviews his notes and textbook, the overwhelming nature of the task becomes apparent. The material builds on concepts he never fully grasped, requiring critical thinking and application skills he hasn't developed due to his surface-level learning approach.

Hours into studying, Sam's thoughts race: "How can I possibly learn all this overnight?", "Why didn't I start earlier?", "Everyone else probably understands this already." Pressure mounts as he realizes memorization won't suffice—he needs to understand and apply complex nursing concepts.

By 11:30 PM, exhausted and stressed, Sam abandons his books and turns to social media, hoping to calm his mind. He contin-

(continued)

ues scrolling until 1:30 AM, then tosses and turns until 3 AM, his sleep disturbed by worry.

The next morning, Sam oversleeps and rushes to the exam, feeling unprepared and overwhelmed. As he faces the complex, application-based questions, he realizes the full impact of his poor time management and study strategies. The cumulative nature of nursing knowledge becomes painfully clear, and he struggles to demonstrate the critical thinking skills required.

For Sam, the accumulation of poor time management and ineffective study habits can lead to a crisis, particularly in a high-stakes situation like a final exam. It emphasizes the unique challenges of nursing education and the importance of developing sustainable study and stress management strategies throughout the semester.

Managing time and keeping performance pressure in check is essential for your nursing school success. The Self-Assessment gave you insight into your time and performance pressures that you can apply to your critical thinking for solutions. Consider making changes to reduce your time pressure if you find yourself like Sam, compromising your performance because of lack of time.

7.4.1 Digital Pressure

Another common pressure faced not just by nursing students but by most everyone in today's culture is digital pressure. Using digital devices to support all aspects of our day is our cultural norm as technology has revolutionized virtually every aspect of our lives. Anywhere you go, a restaurant, a dinner party, a ride on the subway, even a school classroom, you find people giving attention to their devices instead of to the people and places in their surroundings.

Even though evidence suggests our brains are better equipped to learn when we read from a book and handwrite notes on paper, digital resources have even become a part of our educational experience. We cannot escape the digital world in health care. Electronic health records, medical apps, online research databases, e-textbooks, and virtual simulations are just a few examples of the digital tools you're expected to master. While these resources offer unprecedented access to information and learning opportunities, they bring with them new layers of stress.

Digital Stress creates persistent background emotions. Evidence suggests that the constant connectivity that has become our norm is in fact very bad for us, increasing stress and contributing to a host of mental health concerns. This is likely not news to you.

As a nursing student, you are susceptible to digital stress overload in two ways:

- **Multitasking Stress.** Reading from a devise activates different brain pathways than reading from a book but this does not activate stress responses. Multitasking that is common when we are on a device activates the stress response. Scrolling and moving from one task to another contribute to cognitive overload, simultaneously causing hyperarousal and mental fatigue.
- **Notification Stress.** We set notifications for social media, email, messaging apps, and other sources that disrupt our focus, but we are inclined to want these notifications even though we may perceive them as being counterproductive to our well-being. We desire these notifications that provide our brain with moment by moment access to incoming information because we are hooked on them, literally.

Notifications elicit a response in your brain that can be positive or negative as shown in Table 7.4 Digital response.

A positive emotional response is the physiological reward pathway linked to addictive behaviors like gambling. It feels good, and you want more because your brain demands more. This is why it's difficult to just turn your notifica-

7.5 Practical Strategies: Managing Digital Pressure

Table 7.4 Digital response

Positive emotional response	Stressful emotional response
Activates pleasure pathways in the brain triggering release of dopamine	Triggers release of norepinephrine
Feels good	Stimulates sympathetic nervous system
Triggers a desire for more	Detrimental to focus and learning

tions off. You become addicted to the response. So you see, what begins as a positive response ends as a trap. Likewise, activation of the stress response does not contribute to your ability to remain focused and learn. These are compelling reasons for you to assess your digital connectivity and identify where you can make adjustments. Complete the Digital Connectivity Self-Assessment 7.2.

Self-Assessment 7.2: Digital Connectivity

The purpose of this self-assessment activity is to bring awareness to your digital habits, and apply critical thinking to strategies for balancing your digital connectivity and your well-being.

Part 1: Screen Time Analysis

1. Open your device and review your weekly screen time:
   - iPhone: Settings > Screen Time
   - Android: Settings > Digital Well-being
2. Record your findings:
   Total daily average screen time: _____
   Most used apps:
   (a) _____ (hours/day)
   (b) _____ (hours/day)
   (c) _____ (hours/day)
   Number of daily pickups: _____.
   Number of notifications per day: _____.
3. Compare your screen time to the average nursing student (5–7 h/day). How do you compare?

Part 2: Digital Habit Assessment

Table 7.5 Digital habit assessment

Statement	1	2	3	4	5
I check my phone during class					
I study with notifications enabled					
I feel anxious when away from my phone					
I multitask between devices while studying					
I compare myself to others I see on social media					
I use social media during study breaks					
I use devices right before sleeping					
I feel overwhelmed by digital communications					
I have trouble focusing due to digital distractions					
I find myself mindlessly scrolling					
Total					

Rate how often you experience the following on a scale of 1–5
(1 = Never, 5 = Very Often)
Scoring
  40–50: High digital stress impact
  25–39: Moderate digital stress impact
  10–24: Low digital stress impact

Complete Table 7.5 Digital habit assessment.

Are there areas for improvement in managing your digital habits?

Now that you are more aware of your digital habits and the impact of those habits on your well-being and learning, let's look at practical strategies you can use to make changes.

7.5 📝 Practical Strategies: Managing Digital Pressure

Constant digital connectivity is detrimental to our physical and mental well-being. However, in today's world, particularly in health care and education, there is no escaping it. The challenge for you as a nursing student is to set boundaries and create a balance. Developing strategies to manage digital pressure will support both your academic success and your long-term health in your nursing career.

- **Reduce multitasking stress**

Multitasking that is common when we are on a device activates the stress response. Scrolling and moving from one task to another contribute to cognitive overload, simultaneously causing hyperarousal and mental fatigue.

Our brains are just now "wired" for this level of activation. This is why reducing multitasking will improve your focus, enhance your learning, and decrease your overall stress levels.

Be intentional about reducing multitasking first as part of your day-to day-life, and more importantly, when you are learning and studying. Set specific times for checking email and messages, rather than working simultaneously or moving quickly from one to another.

During class and study time, create a distraction-free environment. Turn off notifications, use website blockers, put away your phone, take off your smart watch. Do one activity at a time; in class, attending to the content and learning, during study time, focusing on your studying.

By reducing multitasking, you can improve your focus, enhance your learning, and decrease your overall stress levels.

- **Reduce notification stress**

Even though a notification can elicit a stress response, we are inclined to desire them. The thrill of a notification "what will it be?" is what compels us to want more. This is why putting your phone away or turning off notifications can leave you distracted at first, wondering what you are missing and when you can check!

When you turn off notifications it will take time for your brain to adapt to this change but give it time and intention and you can do it.

While you are in nursing school, there may be notifications you can't turn off. Use your critical thinking skills to determine which notifications you cannot be without, and adjust your device settings to allow only those notifications.

- **Practice mindful consumption**

It is easy to fall into a pattern of mindless consumption, constantly scrolling through social media, news feeds, or entertainment platforms without real engagement or purpose. This passive consumption can lead to information overload, decreased productivity, and increased stress levels.

Mindful consumption involves being intentional and aware of how you interact with digital content. To be mindful, set clear intentions. When you engage with digital content, identify what you want to achieve before you begin scrolling. And remain mindful; focus only on what you are reviewing. Don't multitask (scroll while you are eating, watching TV). Stay attentive while you are on your devices.

If you find it difficult to self-regulate your digital scroll (you may after all, be physiologically addicted to the rewards your brain gets from it!) you can use the time management strategy of time blocking. Allocate specific times for digital scroll and stick to those time frames. You can even set a timer for yourself so you don't get lost in the activity.

By practicing mindful consumption, you can make your digital interactions more purposeful and less stressful. This approach allows you to harness the benefits of digital resources while minimizing their potential negative impacts on your well-being and academic performance.

- **Evaluate your social media use**

Social media platforms like FaceBook, Instagram, X, and TikTok use algorithms to hijack our attention. For nursing students, these platforms can be both a blessing, offering opportunities for networking, sharing information, and staying connected with peers. But they can also be a curse as a source of distraction and stress.

Apply your critical thinking as you consider changes you could make to align your goals (nursing school success) with your activities. Pay attention to how much time you devote to your social media activities, and to how you feel before, during, and after that time. Does it make you feel relaxed and happy or does it leave you with lingering distraction as you think about what you saw.

After you have identified what doesn't support your mental well-being and your time limitations, curate your feeds. You may need to pause or unfollow certain accounts to be more intentional about your social media while you are in nursing school.

Be intentional about recognizing and avoiding the negative thought traps of social media like comparison and fear of missing out (FOMO). Mindfulness will help you recognize and address these negative thought patterns.

You may consider a social media "cleanse" or a complete break from all of your social media. This will be challenging at first, because just like with notifications, you may be physiologically addicted to your social media. A half day "cleanse" will not serve any purpose for you but a longer period of time will allow you to increase your focus on your learning.

Just like addressing digital scroll, social media can be a mindless distraction that interferes with your focus and ability to learn.

It is impossible to avoid digital stress; our devices are not going away. The key is for you to apply your critical thinking to determine which strategies will work best for you to reduce your overall burden of digital stress.

7.5.1 Social Pressure

Social pressure is another external factor that, just like digital stress, is an unavoidable stress that can add to your overall stress burden. Just like other external stressors, social stress activates your norepinephrine stress response and hijacks your ability to remain calm and focused.

Social pressure in nursing school is often intertwined with self-efficacy—your belief in your ability to succeed in specific situations. For many students, particularly those who are shy, introverted, or from diverse cultural backgrounds, social interactions in nursing school can challenge their self-efficacy. This can manifest as difficulty in being assertive, fear of speaking up in class or during clinical rotations, or discomfort in group work.

Moreover, cultural differences can amplify social stress. Students from different cultural backgrounds may find themselves navigating unfamiliar social norms, communication styles, or expectations, which can impact their sense of belonging and willingness to assert themselves.

Take the following social stress self-assessment.

Self-Assessment 7.3: Burden of Social Stress

Social stresses can be both invisible and pervasive. The purpose of this self-assessment activity is to help you recognize how impacted you are by social stress.

Complete Table 7.6 to review your social stress.

As you reflect on your self-assessment results, consider these other aspects of

---

Table 7.6 Social pressure self-assessment

Statement	1	2	3	4	5
I struggle to balance social activities with study time					
I experience stress when working in group projects or study groups					
I feel stressed when I miss out on social events due to academic commitments					
I feel overwhelmed by the social dynamics within my nursing cohort					
I feel burdened by supporting stressed classmates					
I feel stressed when I have to assert myself when interacting with others					
I feel stressed about maintaining relationships outside of nursing school					
Total					

Rate your experience the scale of 1–5
(1 = Never, 5 = Very Often)
Scoring
  7–15: Low social pressure
  16–25: Moderate social pressure
  26–35: High social pressure

personality, culture, and life experience that influence your social stress. Answer the following questions.

1. Reflecting on your self-assessment results, how do you think your level of self-efficacy influences your experience of social stress in nursing school? Consider how being shy, introverted, or assertive might impact your social interactions and stress levels.
2. Consider your support network both inside and outside of nursing school. How can you leverage these relationships to build your self-efficacy and manage social pressure? Are there cultural resources or mentors who could help you navigate the social aspects of nursing school more confidently?

Being aware of these factors will help you as you apply your critical thinking to consider strategies for decreasing the impact of social stress on your well-being while you are in nursing school. These strategies will also support you in your nursing career.

7.6 📝 Practical Strategies: Managing Social Pressure

Managing social pressure is not as straightforward as managing time, performance. and digital pressure. The ways you experience and respond to social pressure are influenced by your personality, life experience, sense of self (self-efficacy), and your culture.

You know yourself better than anyone else, and you know how social stress impacts you. Nursing school is an excellent time to evaluate your social stress response, and to put strategies in place to reduce the impact of social stress on your performance and well-being. In your nursing practice, you will be in a new social environment with social pressure. The skills you learn and incorporate into your habits now will support

not just your nursing school success but support your well-being in your nursing practice.

- **Build self-efficacy**

Self-efficacy is your belief in yourself and your abilities to succeed in social, academic, and work settings. It's not about your actual abilities, but about your confidence in your ability. In nursing school and in nursing practice, strong self-efficacy is a buffer against social pressure.

Some students naturally possess strong self-efficacy, often due to past experiences or supportive environments. However, if you find yourself struggling with self-doubt or feeling overwhelmed by social pressures, know that self-efficacy can be developed and strengthened over time.

To build your self-efficacy, start by recognizing that your belief in yourself is the foundation for self-efficacy. Similar to what was described in Chap. 3 when you believe in your ability to improve your self-efficacy you improve your self-efficacy.

Managing your thoughts is key to improving your self-efficacy. When you hear yourself saying "that person knows more than I do," restate it to a positive "I am just as capable." Refer to Table 4.1 Negative Versus Positive Self-Talk and apply those same principles to your self-efficacy-related self-talk.

Build on your successes as you boost your confidence. You've made it this far! You have accomplished a great deal to get here. You are just as capable as your peers.

Building self-efficacy is a process. Be patient with yourself and acknowledge that growth takes time. As your self-efficacy strengthens, you'll likely find yourself better equipped to handle social pressures and more confident in your abilities as a nursing student.

- **Build a support network**

A strong support network helps reduce social pressure. Connecting with peers who share your values and goals reduces social pressure.

Look for opportunities to connect with classmates who have a growth mindset and positive attitude. Join study groups or form your own with students who share your academic goals. Consider participating in nursing student organizations or volunteer activities where you can meet peers with similar interests.

Your support network doesn't have to be limited to your nursing cohort. Consider including faculty members, academic advisors, students in higher level nursing courses or mentors in your network. These individuals can provide valuable guidance and support as you navigate the social pressures of nursing school.

Building and maintaining a support network requires effort but the benefit of reducing a stressor is a payoff for the effort.

- **Set boundaries**

Setting clear boundaries is helpful for managing social stress. Your social stress self-assessment may have revealed to you social connections that are more draining than supportive. Use your critical thinking as you navigate the social connections you have both within and outside of nursing school.

Establishing boundaries doesn't mean cutting off all social connections. Rather, it's about creating a healthy balance that allows you to engage socially while still prioritizing your academic goals and personal well-being. This might involve limiting time spent with certain individuals, being more selective about which social events you attend, or learning to say no to commitments that interfere with your studies or self-care routine.

Recognize social interactions or commitments that negatively impact you. Do you feel stressed before or after spending time with certain people? Do you consistently sacrifice study time for social activities or feeling pressured to engage in behaviors that don't align with your values or goals? These are important questions to ask yourself as you consider prioritizing your well-being and where to set boundaries.

Setting boundaries is not selfish but a necessary part of reducing your social stress and optimizing your ability to learn and succeed. If you struggle to set boundaries, explore recommendations for increasing your assertiveness.

- **Monitor online social pressure**

While we've discussed digital pressure in terms of device usage and information overload, it's important in this section to address the social pressures that come from online interactions.

As a nursing student, you may feel compelled to present a certain image online—always studying, always succeeding, always balancing your academic and personal life perfectly. This pressure to portray an idealized version of your nursing school experience can be overwhelming and unrealistic. Keep in mind as well that many nursing students who you follow on social media will be striving to project this same image.

As you know social media shows curated highlights of people's lives, not the full picture. Your classmate's post about acing an exam doesn't show the hours of struggle and self-doubt they may have experienced.

Be mindful about your use of social media. Bring awareness to how you feel when you experience a post online. If you notice any feelings that are negative, set boundaries. Consider taking a temporary break from social media, especially during high-stress periods like exam weeks.

Managing social pressure can be daunting but your investment in being mindful about the influence social pressures have on you and incorporating strategies for managing them will help you in nursing school and beyond.

7.6.1 Integrating Stress Management Strategies

Time and performance pressure, digital pressure, and social pressure are common stressors nursing students face and in large part, cannot escape. Implementing strategies to reduce the impact of these stressors will help you create a more balanced and fulfilling nursing school experience.

While you are in nursing school, you have unique stressors that you won't experience in other times of your life. However, stress is ubiquitous; it comes with life and is difficult to escape. Developing healthy stress management skills will support your well-being in your nursing practice.

7.7 📝 Practical Strategies: Managing Stress

The following strategies offer suggestions to help you manage any type of stress. Effective stress management is a life skill to help you maintain balance, focus, and well-being throughout your journey.

- **Apply critical thinking to solve stress overload**

Your critical thinking skills are not just useful for understanding and applying nursing school content. You can use critical thinking to explore and find solutions that will enhance your everyday life. Apply critical thinking to your strategies for identifying stressors, determining which stressors you can address and identifying stress management strategies that will work best for you.

We can get immersed in the routines of our lives, accepting situations and conditions that cause stress but do not serve us. For example, maybe you are in the routine of waiting for your roommate to travel to class together. You're an on time person, your roommate tends to wait until the last minute. Applying critical thinking to this situation, you would ask yourself "how important is it to wait?" Maybe you ponder the implications of arriving to class just before class starts and consider "how does this impact me?" This critical thinking will bring you to the conclusion that you need the extra few minutes before class to get prepared and get the most out of the class session. The stress of not being prepared outweighs the importance of traveling to class with your room-

mate. You decide this is a modifiable stress and elect to travel to class on your own.

Taking a step back to evaluate your routines, and considering how they serve you, can help you reduce stress.

- **Conduct a stress inventory**

Making a list of your external stressors and categorizing them as modifiable or non-modifiable will help you identify stresses that you can control. Here is where you apply your critical thinking to create a plan for reducing or eliminating the stressors you can modify and commit to taking action on making change.

For example, a modifiable stressor might be a "noisy living environment." You could address this by discussing quiet hours with your roommates, investing in noise-canceling headphones, or finding alternative study spaces. An example of a non-modifiable stressor might be "long commute to campus," which you can't eliminate but can manage by using commute time productively (e.g., listening to lecture recordings or study materials).

After identifying your stressors, prioritize addressing the modifiable ones. Create specific, actionable steps for each. Review and update your inventory as your circumstances change throughout nursing school.

- **Adopt a regular routine for relaxing your mind**

Just like committing to a growth mindset changes the structure of your brain, relaxing your mind supports brain structure for decreased impulsivity, reactiveness, and for improved focus. Regular mind relaxation practices have been shown to reduce cortisol levels, increase gray matter density in areas associated with learning and memory.

Review the strategies in Chap. 4 for positive self-talk and relaxing your mind and consider which ones will work best for you. There are many options that include practices such as meditation, deep breathing exercises, progressive muscle relaxation, gratitude, or mindfulness activities. The key is consistency—even short daily practice can yield significant benefits over time.

Remember, the goal is to find techniques that work for you and integrate them into your daily life. This routine will serve as a powerful tool for managing stress.

- **Prioritize your physical health**

Your physical health plays a crucial role in managing stress. The strategies reviewed in Chap. 6 that include getting adequate sleep, balanced nutrition, and physical activity are fundamental to your overall well-being and are powerful tools for stress reduction.

While you may feel too busy or stressed to prioritize these lifestyle habits, keep in mind investing time in these practices will actually improve your ability to handle stress.

- **Know when to seek help**

As mentioned earlier in this chapter, it is important to recognize when you need additional support. When stress overwhelms, seeking help from a counselor or therapist is sometimes a necessary step in maintaining your mental health and academic success.

If you notice significant changes in your ability to concentrate, complete daily tasks, sleep, or appetite, these may be signs that professional help could be beneficial. Isolation from friends and family or thoughts of self-harm are serious indicators of the need for immediate support.

Many nursing students hesitate to seek help, fearing it might be seen as a sign of weakness. However, recognizing when you need support and taking action to get it is a sign of strength and self-awareness. Most colleges and universities offer counseling services to students, often at little or no cost. These professionals are experienced in helping students navigate the unique stressors of academic life.

Seeking help early can prevent small issues from becoming major obstacles to your success and well-being. It's an investment in your mental health that will serve you well throughout your nursing education and career. Don't hesitate to reach out to your school's counseling services or a mental health professional if you feel you need additional support.

Effective stress management is crucial for your success both in nursing school and in nursing practice. By applying critical thinking, conducting regular stress inventories, adopting mind relaxation routines, and prioritizing your physical health, you can build resilience against the various pressures you'll face.

7.8 Conclusion

Stress is an inevitable part of nursing school, but it doesn't have to be a barrier to your success. Not all stress is negative; when managed effectively low levels of stress can even enhance your performance and motivation. The strategies you've learned here for managing time, performance, digital, social, and general stress provide a toolkit for you to individualize your stress management. Applying stress management techniques helps you transform potentially overwhelming stress into a motivating force. Stay attuned to your well-being, adapt your strategies as needed, and don't hesitate to seek support when necessary.

In the next chapter, we will review another common experience for nursing students; anxiety and test anxiety. Just like the toolkit for managing stress that you found in this chapter, you will find a toolkit to help you consider your own anxiety management plan.

Chapter 7 Synthesis Activity: Stress Management Action Plan

In this activity you create a personalized stress management action plan that integrates the various strategies discussed in this chapter.

1. Begin with a stress inventory. List your top three sources of stress in nursing school right now.

(continued)

2. For each stressor on your list, identify two specific strategies from the chapter that you think would be most effective in managing it.
3. Choose one strategy from your list above that you haven't tried before. Describe how you will implement this strategy over the next week. Consider when and how you'll practice and barriers you will have to overcome to implement the strategy.

References

American Psychological Association. (2022, February 14). *What's the difference between stress and anxiety?* https://www.apa.org/topics/stress/anxiety-difference

Heinrich, D., & O'Connell, K. (2024). The effects of mindfulness meditation on nursing students' stress and anxiety levels. *Nursing Education Perspectives, 45*(1), 31–36. https://doi.org/10.1097/01. NEP.0000000000001159

Lazarus, R. S. (1984). *Stress, appraisal, and coping* (Vol. 464). Springer.

Turner, K., & McCarthy, V. L. (2017). Stress and anxiety among nursing students: A review of intervention strategies in literature between 2009 and 2015. *Nurse Education in Practice, 22*, 21–29. https://doi.org/10.1016/j.nepr.2016.11.002

Uysal, N., & Çalışkan, B. B. (2022). The effects of mindfulness-based stress reduction on mindfulness and stress levels of nursing students during first clinical experience. *Perspectives in Psychiatric Care, 58*(4), 2639–2645. https://doi.org/10.1111/ppc.13104

Windle, S., & Musselman, E. (2022). Evaluation of a brief stress management workshop for incoming nursing students. *Holistic Nursing Practice, 36*(3), 128–138. https://doi.org/10.1097/HNP.0000000000000510

Manage Your Anxiety and Conquer Test Anxiety

8

> *Anxiety is like a rocking chair; it gives you something to do but doesn't get you very far.*
> —Jodi Picoult

8.1 Introduction

Anxiety is a common experience for nursing students, often intensified by the rigorous demands of nursing school. As noted in Chap. 7, stress and anxiety are often used interchangeably, and while related, they are distinct experiences with different causes and manifestations. Strategies for managing stress are reviewed in that chapter. This chapter focuses on understanding anxiety, particularly in the context of nursing education, and provides strategies to manage both general anxiety and test anxiety.

▶ **By the end of this chapter you will be able to:**
1. Differentiate between stress and anxiety, understanding their unique impacts on learning.
2. Identify personal triggers and symptoms of anxiety.
3. Apply practical strategies to manage general anxiety in nursing school.
4. Implement techniques to reduce test anxiety and improve exam performance.
5. Develop a personalized anxiety management plan that supports well-being and academic success.

8.2 Anxiety and Stress

Anxiety and stress are related issues. This comparison, reviewed in Chap. 7, noted that even though these terms are often used interchangeably, and each can impact your ability to focus, learn, and apply critical thinking, they are different from one another.

Stress is a result of external factors, some of which can be controlled as reviewed in the Practical Strategies section in Chap. 7. It is important to note that some low levels of stress can actually help us to be more productive.

Anxiety on the other hand is seldom productive, and results from internal, not external factors.

In Table 8.1 you see the comparison between stress and anxiety that was presented in Chap. 7.

As a nursing student you are likely to have both stress and some level of anxiety. Even if you didn't experience anxiety before nursing school, it has been documented that nursing school elicits anxiety (Quinn & Peters, 2017; Robinson et al., 2024).

This chapter focuses on managing anxiety to enhance your overall learning experience and addressing test anxiety to improve your performance on exams. Both aspects are crucial for your success in nursing school.

© The Author(s), under exclusive license to Springer Nature Switzerland AG 2025
C. Thompson, *Nursing School, NCLEX and Career Transition Success*,
https://doi.org/10.1007/978-3-031-85538-2_8

Table 8.1 Characteristics of stress and anxiety

Stress	Anxiety
Body's response to specific demands or challenges	A persistent feeling of worry or fear
Can be positive (eustress) or negative (distress)	More negative than positive
Typically tied to identifiable external factors or events	Often not tied to a specific external trigger and persists in the absence of immediate stressors
Can motivate performance or overwhelm when chronic	May involve anticipation of future threats
May subside when the stressor is removed	Tends to be long-lasting

If you suffer from an anxiety disorder, this chapter does not replace care or treatment from a mental health care provider. You need to continue with that care and treatment. Nursing school is not the time to make drastic changes or stop treatments that have been working for you.

8.3 Anxiety and Brain-Based Learning

Anxiety activates the sympathetic nervous system, which prepares the body for "fight or flight" responses. This results in several physiological effects, including increased heart rate, rapid breathing, and heightened alertness. "Fight or flight" responses are beneficial in short-term, immediate-threat situations, like when you are walking in the woods and you see a bear. The sympathetic nervous system activation allows you to run from that bear. Heart rate and breathing increase to improve flow of oxygenated blood to the large muscle groups allowing you to go as fast as possible to outrun the bear. In this fight or flight moment, learning about the experience and remembering details is not important for your survival.

This sympathetic nervous system activation is counterproductive to your learning, impacting several parts of your brain.

- **Amygdala activation.** Activation of the amygdala signals the hypothalamus to release stress hormones like adrenaline and cortisol. This activation interferes with the brains' ability to process new information and form memories. This explains why some people are not able to remember a traumatic event such as an accident. The survival mechanism overrides memory consolidation.

- **Prefrontal cortex suppression.** Anxiety impairs the functioning of the prefrontal cortex, reducing its efficiency. This leads to difficulties in focusing, processing information, and retaining new knowledge. As the prefrontal cortex is less effective, the ability to think critically and solve problems diminishes.

- **Hippocampus impairment.** The hippocampus has a role in forming and retrieving memories. Anxiety can reduce the volume of the hippocampus, impairing its ability to function effectively. This shrinkage can lead to difficulties in learning new information and recalling previously learned material, severely impacting academic performance.

- **Neurotransmitter imbalance.** Anxiety affects the balance of neurotransmitters, such as serotonin and dopamine, which modulate for mood, motivation, and cognitive functions. Imbalances in these neurotransmitters can lead to mood disorders, decreased motivation, and cognitive impairments, further hindering the learning process and overall mental health.

Now you can see why anxiety impacts your ability to learn and be successful in nursing school and why "test anxiety" has a huge impact on test performance. Anxiety interferes with your ability to learn, process, integrate new learning, remember what you learned, apply critical thinking, and recall learned information.

You can complete an anxiety screening tool to determine your general levels of anxiety.

Table 8.2 GAD-7

Over the last 2 weeks how often have you been bothered by the following problems?	Not at all	Several days	More than half the days	Nearly every day
1. Feeling nervous, anxious or on edge	0	1	2	3
2. Not being able to stop or control worrying	0	1	2	3
3. Worrying too much about different things	0	1	2	3
4. Trouble relaxing	0	1	2	3
5. Being so restless that it's hard to sit still	0	1	2	3
6. Becoming easily annoyed or irritable	0	1	2	3
7. Feeling afraid, as if something might happen	0	1	2	3
Total score (add results from each column)				

Self-Assessment 8.1: Anxiety Screening

You may be familiar with the GAD-7 (Spitzer et al., 2006), which is a screening tool for anxiety (Generalized Anxiety Disorder.) It is a valid and reliable tool that is used in clinical practice for assessment of anxiety. By completing the GAD on Table 8.2, you can see how many common symptoms you have and where you might fall in the range of anxiety; from mild to severe.

Choose one answer for each of the seven questions:

Your total score is a guide to how severe your anxiety disorder may be

0 to 4 = mild anxiety
5 to 9 = moderate anxiety
10 to 14 = moderately severe anxiety
15 to 21 = severe anxiety

The GAD-7 is a screening tool, and as with all screening tools, it does not diagnose anxiety disorder. If your results (10 or higher) suggest you might be experiencing severe anxiety you should consider pursuing diagnosis and treatment from a mental health provider. Your college or university should have mental health resources for you to access.

8.3.1 Cumulative Anxiety in Nursing School

The pressures that are a part of life (digital stress, time stress) as well as the pressures in nursing school (performance pressure, peer pressure) can contribute to anxiety. Being aware of these pressures and using proactive strategies to reduce your susceptibility to anxiety from these factors will support your success.

8.4 Practical Strategies: Managing Anxiety in Nursing School

Many of the practical strategies for managing stress that were included in Chap. 7 apply here in regard to managing anxiety while you are in nursing school. Others on this list are specific to managing anxiety.

- **Keep up with your care**

As noted in the introduction to this chapter, if you have been diagnosed with an anxiety disorder, the recommendations in this chapter are not for the purpose of replacing your treatment regimen. Now is **not** the time to discontinue treatment that has been supporting you. Continue care with your mental health provider, continue prescribed medication, and behavioral interventions that have worked for you.

- **Know when to seek help and seek help when you know you need it**

Even if you're already under care for anxiety, there may be times during nursing school when you need additional support. If you've never been in care for an anxiety disorder, the stresses of nursing school can lead to greater anxiety that may require professional help.

The strategies in this chapter can help you manage anxiety but it is important to recognize when your anxiety is overwhelming or interfering with your well-being and your studies. Signs that it's time to seek professional help include persistent worry that's hard to control, difficulty concentrating or sleeping, physical symptoms like rapid heartbeat or upset stomach, avoiding classes or clinical rotations due to anxiety, or feeling hopeless.

Most colleges and universities offer counseling services for students, often at low or no cost. These professionals are experienced in helping students navigate the unique stressors of academic life, including those specific to nursing programs. Don't hesitate to reach out to your school's counseling center or student health services. They can provide tools and support tailored to your needs.

Seeking help is a sign of strength, not weakness. It shows you're committed to your well-being and success in nursing school. Being proactive about your mental health will not only help you manage your anxiety but also prepare you for the demands of your future nursing career.

- **Reduce modifiable stressors**

While stress and anxiety have distinct characteristics as outlined in Table 8.1, Characteristics of Stress and Anxiety, they are also interrelated. As your stress increases, so does your anxiety. This relationship is particularly important to understand in the context of nursing school, where many stressors are unavoidable.

Review the practical strategies in Chap. 7 and prioritize reducing external stresses that can be addressed while you are in nursing school. Not all stressors can be eliminated, but many can be managed or reduced.

Several stressors you can evaluate and reduce are reviewed in other chapters in this book. Consider your time management, are you over-committed and are there changes you could consider as outlined in Chap. 5. Do you have a healthy approach to planning your academic activities that allow you to adopt a growth mindset approach to support your learning? This is reviewed in Chap. 3.

As you review the content, apply your critical thinking to determine how you can adjust your lifestyle to support your ability to manage anxiety during this time you are in nursing school.

- **Incorporate a daily practice for relaxing your mind**

As discussed in Chaps. 4 and 7, committing to regular practice for calming your mind is essential for managing anxiety. Meditation, mindfulness, gratitude, prayer, guided imagery, progressive relaxation, journaling, and yoga are just a few examples of practices for mind relaxation.

None of these practices are as effective as one time intervention as they are when incorporated into your daily routine. This is because the practices, when done consistently, change the structure of your brain, making it more difficult for anxiety pathways to predominate.

If you are not in a practice of mind relaxation, it will be challenging at first, because your brain is not wired for relaxation. Committing to the practice is vital to your ability to make the practice effective. As you begin, start slow. If you've never meditated, you will find the first 60 s session of a meditation practice grueling. Give it time, as you commit to it on a daily basis you'll find your brain aligning itself to the new practice. As soon as you go to your quiet space, you'll be able to feel your brain, and your body, calming. This calm is the reflection of the new pathways you have created that will support your ongoing ability to be calm.

Explore various strategies to find which works best for you. There are apps to support your practice, some that are free and some with minimal costs. Set your goal to find a technique that works for you and integrate it into your daily life. Just as

8.4 Practical Strategies: Managing Anxiety in Nursing School

this practice is a powerful stress management tool, it is a powerful anxiety management tool.

- **Make movement a priority**

Physical activity is a powerful tool for managing anxiety. As a nursing student, you might feel you don't have time for exercise, but even short bursts of activity can significantly reduce anxiety levels.

Exercise releases endorphins, often called "feel-good" hormones, which can improve mood and reduce anxiety. It also helps to decrease muscle tension, lowering the physical symptoms of anxiety.

For nursing students, incorporating exercise can be as simple as taking a brisk walk between classes or doing a quick yoga session before studying. These activities not only reduce anxiety but can also improve focus and retention of information, supporting your brain-based learning.

The goal isn't to become an athlete. Just try to move your body regularly. Find activities you enjoy to make your physical activity something to look forward to rather than to dread. The key is consistency rather than intensity.

- **Sleep Sleep Sleep**

Getting enough sleep is essential for managing anxiety and supporting your learning in nursing school. It's a known fact that not getting enough sleep makes anxiety worse. When you're tired, your brain is less able to handle stress and worry.

Aim for 6–8 h of sleep each night. This might seem hard with your busy schedule, but making sleep a priority will help reduce your anxiety and make your awake time more productive for learning.

Strategies for better sleep are outlined in Chap. 6. If you find it hard to get 6–8 h of sleep, review those detailed tips. They can help you create better sleep habits. However, if anxiety is keeping you awake even when you try these strategies, it's important to seek help. Talk to a mental health provider. They can offer support and additional tools to manage anxiety that's interfering

with your sleep. Getting professional help when you need it is a sign of strength, not weakness.

- **Fuel your body and brain**

What you eat plays a big role in managing anxiety. Poor nutrition can make anxiety worse, while a balanced diet can help keep you calm and focused.

Eat regular, balanced meals throughout the day. Skipping meals can lead to low blood sugar, which can feel like anxiety and make actual anxiety worse. Keep healthy snacks on hand for long study sessions or clinical rotations.

Strategies for maintaining a healthy diet are also detailed in Chap. 6. If you're struggling to eat well with your busy schedule, review those tips. They can help you make better food choices even when you're short on time.

If your eating habits are being affected by anxiety, or if you're using food to cope with anxiety, it's important to seek help. Talk to a health care provider or a nutritionist. They can offer guidance on using nutrition to support your mental health. Taking care of your body is just as important as taking care of your mind when you are working to reduce your anxiety.

- **Stay connected, not overwhelmed**

Social connections are important for managing anxiety, but finding the right balance is key. Isolation can make anxiety worse but overcommitting to social activities can lead to stress which makes anxiety worse.

Maintain meaningful connections without overwhelming your schedule. This might mean joining a study group, having a "study buddy" for mutual support, or scheduling regular check-ins with family or close friends. Participating in nursing student organizations can be beneficial, but limit your involvement to what feels manageable.

Quality of social connections often matters more than quantity. A few strong, supportive relationships can be more beneficial for managing anxiety than a large number of superficial ones.

Don't be afraid to set boundaries. The right balance between meaningful connections that support your well-being and overcommitment will help you manage anxiety.

- **Be a good student**

Being well-prepared for classes, exams, and clinical rotations will reduce anxiety. The Student Behavior section in Chap. 6 reviews strategies for prioritizing academic work, being prepared for class, and scheduling time for content review to support brain-based learning.

Adopting these strategies will improve your ability to succeed, which will boost your confidence and reduce your anxiety about academic performance.

Strategies for preparation and effective studying will also be crucial in managing test anxiety, which are reviewed in the next section. Developing strong study habits reduces general anxiety and lays the foundation for better performance and reduced anxiety during exams.

In this section, you have a toolkit of strategies you can use to decrease your overall anxiety while you are in nursing school. Taking steps to adopt these strategies improves your brain-based learning and allows you to apply your critical thinking and maintain a growth mindset throughout your learning journey.

8.5 Test Anxiety in Nursing School

In the previous section we reviewed how anxiety impacts your learning and performance in nursing school. Here we will focus on a specific type of anxiety that most nursing students report—test anxiety (McCormick & Lamberson, 2024). Understanding test anxiety, how it differs from general anxiety, and strategies to manage it will help you perform at your best when it matters most, on exam day.

In this section, the words "test" and "exam" are used interchangeably.

8.6 Test Anxiety

Unlike general anxiety, which may be a constant background presence throughout nursing school, test anxiety typically surfaces in response to exams or evaluations.

Test anxiety is common among nursing students. When talking with your instructors about test anxiety, you may hear this advice; "Being prepared for the test is the best way to manage test anxiety." While being well-prepared is a powerful tool to combat anxiety, it's important to recognize that if general anxiety is already present, it can amplify test-specific fears.

Table 8.3 outlines two types of anxiety students may experience related to test-taking.

Understanding the type of test anxiety you're experiencing can help you create a plan for addressing it.

8.6.1 The Physiology of Test Anxiety

Both types of test anxiety trigger the "fight or flight" response in your body. As reviewed in the previous section in this chapter, this response is designed to help us escape immediate danger, like outrunning a predator. It is not helpful in a testing environment.

Recall that in "fight or flight" various areas of your brain including the amygdala, prefrontal cortex, hippocampus, as well as your neurotransmitters are impacted. These changes impair your ability to recall information, retrieve stored knowledge, think clearly, and make connections. Basically, the processes that support critical

Table 8.3 Types of test anxiety

Preparation test anxiety	Emotional test anxiety
Performance anxiety stemming from ineffective time management or study skills	Fear, worry, and/or dread stemming from underlying general anxiety

8.6.2 Preparation Test Anxiety

This is where your instructors are correct; adequate preparation for your exams will address preparation test anxiety. These are many aspects of test preparation for you to consider. Complete the Test Preparation Practices given in Table 8.4 as you explore your own preparation test anxiety.

thinking are put on hold while you are experiencing anxiety, limiting your ability to demonstrate your knowledge when you take an exam.

The sympathetic nervous system response also triggers changes in your body. If you experience test anxiety you know how this feels; your heart races, your hands sweat, and feel nauseous, and your thoughts become disorganized. Just like the impact on your brain, this body response impacts your test performance. These symptoms create a feedback loop that reinforces anxiety.

Understanding these reactions helps you better appreciate why managing anxiety is essential for your best exam performance. Let's review strategies to help you address both types of test anxiety; preparation and emotional test anxiety.

Self-Assessment 8.2: Test Preparation Practices

Complete the following self-assessment to assess your habits for exam preparation. Answer each question based on your typical behavior when preparing for a test (Table 8.4).

Your total score reflects test preparation practices that impact test preparedness

21–30 = strong test preparation practices
11–20 = effective preparation practices with room for improvement
1–10 = weak preparation practices that contribute to test preparedness

Reflect on your results. Which areas of your test preparation could be improved? How can you apply the strategies reviewed in previous chapters of the book to strengthen your test preparation?

Your self-assessment most likely reveals what you already suspected if you experience test anxiety because you find yourself not feeling prepared on exam day.

Managing test preparation really does come down to what your instructors advise "be prepared for the test." You can use the strategies out-

Table 8.4 Test preparation strategies

Statement	Never (0)	Sometimes (1)	Often (2)	Always (3)
I include in my schedule time to review the material covered in class right after class				
I break my study sessions into manageable chunks instead of cramming all at once				
I use active learning strategies when I am preparing for class and reviewing content				
I study each day in the week leading up to an exam rather than cramming the day before				
When I study I do so in an environment free of distractions (e.g., noise, social media interruptions)				
I prioritize getting adequate sleep				
I use a planner or calendar to organize my time				
I have a daily practice of mind relaxation strategies to manage my stress, anxiety and improve my learning				
I revisit challenging material multiple times rather than avoiding it				
I commit to critical thinking in my learning				

lined in previous chapters in this book to improve your critical thinking and learning as you prepare for exams and the rewards will pay off on exam day.

8.6.3 Emotional Test Anxiety

Emotional test anxiety can be a learned response that may not be entirely grounded in reality. It may stem from past negative experiences or an ingrained fear of failure that becomes a conditioned response during exams. Unlike preparation test anxiety, which can be alleviated through effective study habits, emotional anxiety requires addressing underlying fears and managing thought patterns.

Managing emotional test anxiety starts with recognizing that anxiety is a highly individualized experience. Your level of anxiety will depend on various factors, including your underlying general anxiety, past experiences, and personality. The strategies presented here are intended to help you manage test-related anxiety, but they are not meant to replace prescribed treatment or mental health care if you are experiencing a diagnosed anxiety disorder.

It is difficult to completely eliminate test anxiety; test day nerves are bound to occur, particularly in nursing school where exams can have high stakes for you; passing or failing a course. Managing your baseline anxiety will support your ability to address your anxiety on test day.

8.7 📝Practical Strategies: Managing Test Anxiety

Managing test anxiety will help you avoid the sympathetic nervous system response that interferes with your ability to stay focused and use critical thinking to apply what you have learned to the test questions. The following strategies will further support your ability to remain calm and focused to perform your best.

- **Address negative self-talk**

Self-talk management is an important starting point for addressing test anxiety. Positive self-talk does not replace being prepared for a test, but it is a valuable tool for addressing performance test anxiety. Negative self-talk intensifies emotional anxiety, while positive, constructive self-talk can help reduce it.

Refer to the practical strategies outlined in Chap. 4 to address and improve your self-talk.

Be intentional about maintaining your positive self-talk as you prepare for exams and when you take exams. Prior to the exam, replace negative thoughts such as "I might not know enough" with positives "I am prepared and calm." During the exam, replace negative thoughts such as "I always do bad on select all that apply questions" with "I have to read carefully and do my best."

- **Reduce your overall stress**

You can reduce your baseline anxiety levels by reducing modifiable stressors.

When you are dealing with test anxiety, you can't make changes on test day to alter your experience of test anxiety. Managing test anxiety requires the integration of strategies for improving your overall well-being. As noted in other parts of this book, making these changes will improve your test anxiety, improve your test performance, and give you skills that carry over to all aspects of your learning to think like a nurse, and your ability to function with a high level of well-being in your nursing practice. Controlling baseline anxiety leads to less test day anxiety.

- **Swap out all night cramming for sleep**

As noted throughout this book, sleep is your basic building block for reducing anxiety and optimal test performance. When you are adopting student behaviors for brain-based learning, you're not leaving long stretches of studying until the night before an exam. In all cases, a good night of sleep is a better option for addressing test

8.7 Practical Strategies: Managing Test Anxiety

anxiety than an all-night or even late-night cramming session. Good sleep is essential both for processing your learning and reducing your anxiety.

- **Provide food for your brain**

Elements of nutrition that support learning are reviewed in Chap. 6. Separate from that, it is important to remember that a consistent glucose level throughout a test provides energy for your brain. Protein and fat are digested slowly and provide a gradual release of glucose into your bloodstream. A high carbohydrate meal leads to a rapid spike and subsequent drop in blood sugar which can cause you to lose focus.

On test day, prioritize time for a balanced meal with protein and fat in advance of your exam. This provides your brain with "fuel" for thinking and application of your learning, and prevents the anxiety your body experiences when your blood glucose level drops.

- **Know the rules and be prepared to follow them**

Unfortunately, in many nursing programs the exam rules vary from course to course, making your work as a nursing student more challenging as you are required to know rules for each instructor. You will need to review exam guidelines before test day.

For online exams, make sure your testing environment meets all requirements such as proper lighting. Have required software installed and working properly on your device. Many testing platforms offer practice tests or tutorials— use these to familiarize yourself with the system. Learn how to navigate between questions, flag items for review, and submit your answers. If your exam requires remote proctoring with camera monitoring, test your equipment ahead of time. Do a trial run of your technology setup, including your internet connection.

For in-person exams, be prepared to follow the rules about personal items like cell phones,

smartwatches, water bottles, and backpacks. If items are to be stored outside the exam room, prepare for that in advance. Last minute disruptions caused by not being prepared can derail your calm and trigger anxiety.

As part of the review of rules for preparing, make sure you know the time allotted for the test to pace yourself accordingly.

If you are using accommodations for testing, follow the instructions in the syllabus for notifying the instructor and familiarize yourself with accommodation center location and rules.

- **Arrive early**

This is obvious but important to include because in terms of test anxiety, a last minute scramble to the test produces anxiety. Give yourself plenty of time (15–20 min) to arrive at the exam location. This allows plenty of time for unexpected last minute delays. Use this time to practice calming techniques and focus your mind on the task ahead.

- **Choose your company wisely**

For in-person tests, when you arrive in advance, you will be around classmates who will be discussing the exam. Avoid groups who are discussing how stressed they are. If necessary, find a quiet space to maintain your calm. If removing yourself from negative pretest circles of friends creates social pressure for you, refer to the practical strategies for addressing social pressure reviewed in Chap. 7.

- **Chew gum**

Believe it or not, gum chewing has been associated with decreased test anxiety among nursing students in one small study (Yaman et al., 2019). Of course, you'd want to chew sugarless gum, and in this study, students who practiced chewing gum for a few minutes a day and during testing had improved academic performance and reduced self-reported anxiety compared to students who did not chew gum. Worth a try.

- ### Practice relaxation techniques

Relaxation techniques are reviewed in various chapters in this book. Many methods have been shown to be effective. These include deep breathing, mindfulness, prayer, progressive muscle relaxation, imagery, aromatherapy, or mantras to name a few of the most popular. A relaxation technique that works for you activates your parasympathetic nervous system helping you to stay calm. You can use that to keep yourself calm before the test, and during testing when you notice anxiety.

The most important thing about this is incorporating a relaxation practice into your regular routine. This will help to reprogram your brain for the calming response that you desire. If you haven't reprogrammed your brain for this, implementing something new on test day is not likely to be effective for addressing your test anxiety.

- ### Manage your response to your environment

Know what distracts you and prepare to minimize those distractions during exams.

For in-person testing, choose your seat based on your needs for reducing distraction. If movement or activity catches your attention, select a spot away from windows, doors, or high-traffic areas. Some students prefer to sit at the front where they can't see other test-takers, while others do better in the back where they have a view of the whole room. Know what works for you and position yourself accordingly.

Don't let other students' actions derail your concentration. If someone finishes early, resist the urge to compare yourself. Use positive self-talk; instead of thinking "I must be doing something wrong if they're done and I'm only halfway through," say instead "I'm taking the time I need to read each question carefully and demonstrate my knowledge." Your pace is your pace—what matters is that you're giving each question the attention it deserves.

For online testing, set up in a quiet space where you won't be interrupted. Turn off phone notifications, close unnecessary browser tabs, and remove potential distractions from your workspace. Consider using noise-canceling headphones if you can't eliminate background noises.

When you do encounter a distraction, use the relaxation and calming techniques to refocus.

- ### Use the five step method for test taking

This essential test taking strategy will help you to maintain focus and avoid missing questions because of reading errors.

Step 1: Read the question carefully
Focus on what the question is specifically asking. Identify keywords that focus your attention on what is being asked and provide cues to what the answer might be.
Don't read the answers yet!
Step 2: Analyze the question
Here is where you are using your critical thinking. Don't read the answers yet! Review what the question is asking; What nursing concept is being tested? What relevant nursing priorities should be considered? What cues are provided in the question? At this point you may even want to predict which answer you would be looking for.
Step 3: Read each answer option
As you carefully read each answer option one at a time, consider for each a yes/no/maybe. Even if you read an answer you choose at "yes" don't select it until you have read every answer option.
Step 4: Select your answer
Step 5: Move to the next question
Don't change your answer unless you are certain. Your first instinct is more likely to be the correct answer than a second guess. If you are uncertain of an answer and are permitted to go back over questions, flag it for review after you have completed the exam.

This five step method takes practice in order for it to become your habit on test day. Use it when you take practice tests to make it second nature on exam day.

- **Avoid "after test" anxiety**

When you have completed an exam, resist the urge to join classmates' discussions about answers to exam questions. These conversations rarely reduce anxiety and often increase it, especially if you learn you answered differently from your peers. Instead of participating in the "post-mortem" analysis of the test, take a few minutes for yourself. Use positive self-talk to acknowledge that you did your best and the outcome is now beyond your control.

Accept exam results with a growth mindset. Apply your critical thinking to your self-evaluation of your exam preparation and performance, and adjust your study strategies for the next exam rather than allowing it to fuel anxiety about future tests.

Effective exam day preparation is the end result of your efforts to manage both performance and emotional anxiety. Being well-prepared for the exam and reducing your baseline anxiety lays a foundation for success. The exam day strategies serve as the final touch, enhancing your ability to perform at your best when it matters most.

These strategies aren't just for your nursing school exams. They will serve you well as you prepare for and take the NCLEX exam. This is the exam where you will reach your ultimate goal: becoming a nurse. Addressing test anxiety throughout nursing school will give you the tools to perform your best on that most critical exam.

8.8 Conclusion

Anxiety significantly impacts brain function, particularly in areas critical for learning and performance, which is why test preparation, managing baseline anxiety and test day planning are keys for exam success. The strategies discussed in this chapter support optimal brain function, allowing your prefrontal cortex to engage in critical thinking, your hippocampus to effectively retrieve and consolidate memories, and your neurotransmit-

ters to maintain balance for better cognitive performance. While some anxiety is normal, especially on test day, you can prevent it from becoming overwhelming.

In the next chapter, we'll explore how Artificial Intelligence can serve as a powerful supplement to your learning toolkit, offering new ways to reinforce your understanding and practice critical thinking skills without replacing the work you do to perform your best.

> **Chapter 8 Synthesis Learning Activity: Anxiety Management Plan**
> This activity is designed to help apply what you learned in this chapter to create a personalized anxiety management toolkit by reflecting on past experiences and applying strategies learned in this chapter.
>
> 1. Reflect on your past exam experiences to complete Table 8.5.
> 2. Consider new strategies, and write your ideas in Table 8.6.
> 3. Outline a step-by-step routine for the night before and morning of an exam, incorporating at least one strategy for reducing baseline anxiety.
> 4. Post-exam reflection: Write down two questions you'll ask yourself after your next exam to assess the effectiveness of your anxiety management strategies.

Table 8.5 Strategies for staying calm

Strategy I have used to stay calm during tests	Evaluation—was it effective and if not, why?
1.	
2.	
3.	

Table 8.6 Strategies to try

Strategy to try	Why I think it will work for me
1.	
2.	

References

McCormick, S., & Lamberson, J. (2024). Interventions for test anxiety in nursing students: A literature review. *Teaching & Learning in Nursing, 19*(2), e404–e411. https://doi.org/10.1016/j.teln.2024.01.005

Quinn, B. L., & Peters, A. (2017). Strategies to reduce nursing student test anxiety: A literature review. *Journal of Nursing Education, 56*(3), 145–151. https://doi.org/10.3928/01484834-20170222-05

Robinson, L. A., Short, P. R., & Frugé, A. D. (2024). Sleep quality and interoception are associated with generalized anxiety in baccalaureate nursing students: A cross-sectional study. *Nursing Reports, 14*(2), 1184–1192. https://doi.org/10.3390/nursrep14020090

Spitzer, R. L., Kroenke, K., Williams, J. B. W., & Löwe, B. (2006). A brief measure for assessing generalized anxiety disorder: The GAD-7. *Archives of Internal Medicine, 166*(10), 1092–1097.

Yaman, S., Ayaz, A., & Bayrak, K. (2019). Effect of chewing gum on stress, anxiety, depression, self-focused attention, and academic success: A randomized controlled study. *Stress and Health, 35*(4), 441–446. https://doi.org/10.1002/smi.2872

Using AI to Support Your Learning

9

AI is a tool. The choice about how it gets deployed is ours.

—*Oren Etzioni (CEO: Allen Institute for Artificial Intelligence)*

9.1 Introduction

Artificial intelligence (AI) has rapidly become a part of our everyday lives, often without us even realizing it. When you search for information online, scroll through social media, or ask your smartphone for directions, you're interacting with AI. It's evolving rapidly and woven into the fabric of our digital world, shaping how we access information and make decisions. In this chapter, we'll explore how you can harness AI to support your nursing education while maintaining academic integrity. We'll dive into practical applications, ethical considerations, and strategies for using AI as an ally in mastering nursing knowledge and skills.

▶ **By the end of this chapter you will be able to:**
1. Evaluate ethical implications of using AI in nursing education identifying appropriate that enhance learning without compromising academic integrity.
2. Develop effective AI prompts.
3. Demonstrate responsible use of AI as a supplement to, not a replacement for critical thinking and problem-solving skills.

4. Analyze AI-generated responses for accuracy and relevance to nursing practice.
5. Integrate AI tools to reinforce understanding of nursing concepts, prepare for exams, and navigate the challenges of nursing school.

9.2 AI in Nursing and Health Care

Just as AI is present in our everyday lives, it is being used in nursing and health care. As you progress through your clinical experiences, you'll see and work with AI tools that supplement and enhance aspects of care. Numerous examples of how AI is being integrated in health care settings have been reported in the literature (Alowais et al., 2023; Douthit et al., 2022; Foronda et al., 2024) and will continue to expand at unprecedented speed.

- **Early fall prevention**: AI is used to monitor client movements for early detection of falls. These systems detect early indications of changes that precede a client's attempt to get

© The Author(s), under exclusive license to Springer Nature Switzerland AG 2025
C. Thompson, *Nursing School, NCLEX and Career Transition Success*,
https://doi.org/10.1007/978-3-031-85538-2_9

out of bed. These systems are capable of identifying movement patterns before a human "sitter" would see them and before a bed alarm detects the client getting out of bed.

- **Electronic health record (EHR) data entry**: AI can record nursing actions and populate accurate data into the Electronic Health Record (EHR). These tools go beyond simple data entry, capable of documenting nurse–client interactions, client subjective data, and nursing interventions.
- **Medication administration**: AI tools assist nurses in medication administration by providing real-time dosage calculations, checking for potential drug interactions or allergies, and ensuring that the right medication is administered to the right client at the right time. I know what you're thinking—why do I have to learn drug and dosage calculations? You need to know these in order to provide safe care in settings where these tools are not available. In addition, what about a disaster or power outage? AI will not replace nurses' needing to know how to do this!
- **Predictive analytics for client care**: Client data can be analyzed to predict potential health complications. For instance, AI can identify risk for developing pressure ulcers, sepsis, or other conditions, allowing nurses to take proactive measures.
- **Remote monitoring**: AI devices and wearables continuously monitor clients' vital signs, sending alerts to nurses when important changes are detected.
- **Diagnosis:** AI tools are increasingly being used to identify patterns in symptoms or imaging that could indicate specific conditions faster and, in some cases, more accurately, than humans.
- **Client engagement and education**: AI powered Chatbots and virtual assistants provide clients with personalized health information, reminders for medication or appointments, and answers to health-related questions. Some studies have even shown AI Chatbot responses are more compassionate and caring than responses from nurses and providers!

- **Language interpretation**: AI language models facilitate communication when clients speak different languages and an interpreter is not available. Instead of waiting for a human or virtual interpreter, AI can be readily available in a handheld device.
- **Simulation education:** AI virtual reality tools are used in simulation to create realistic and adaptive learning scenarios to enhance education.

These are just a few examples of early AI applications. Let's explore how AI can support your educational journey, helping you to better understand complex concepts, practice critical thinking, and prepare for your future career.

9.3   AI in Nursing Education

AI has sparked both excitement and concern in education. Since the launch of ChatGPT in November 2022, many discussions about AI in academia have focused on detecting its use in student work and preventing cheating (Bumbach, 2024). However, AI's potential in education extends far beyond these concerns. When used responsibly, AI can be a powerful tool to enhance learning.

From clarifying complex concepts to generating practice scenarios, when used in nursing school, AI offers innovative ways to reinforce your understanding and critical thinking skills (Simms, 2025).

AI is a broad term that encompasses all aspects of artificial intelligence. The AI reviewed in this chapter is referred to as a Large Language Model (LLM), which generates text responses based on review of what has been written in books, magazines, on the internet, and other written language sources. You can also use AI to generate images and videos. We will include examples of how generative text responses or images can support your learning.

There are several AI products you can access for free and others that are low cost. For the examples in this chapter, we will use ChatGPT, which was the first LLM available for public use. Others that were available early on when AI launched to the public include Bard, Microsoft Bing, Apple AI, and Claude.

Before we dive deeper into how to use AI effectively in your nursing education, let's take a moment to reflect on your current understanding and use of AI. This self-assessment will help you identify your strengths and areas for improvement when it comes to incorporating AI into your studies.

By evaluating your current AI skills and knowledge, you'll be better equipped to make the most of the strategies and tips we'll discuss in this chapter. Remember, there's no "right" or "wrong" level of AI proficiency. The AI in Nursing Education Self-Assessment 9.1 will help you understand where you are and where you might want to focus your efforts as you learn to leverage AI.

Self-Assessment 9.1: AI in Nursing Education

On a scale of 1–10 rate your agreement with each of the following (Table 9.1)

Based on your AI self-assessment responses, identify:

1. Two areas where you feel confident in your AI usage
2. Two areas where you'd like to improve your AI skills
3. One specific goal for incorporating AI more effectively into your nursing studies

Now that you've assessed your current AI skills and knowledge, it's important to consider the ethical implications of using AI in your nursing education. As you work to improve your AI proficiency and integrate it into your studies, understanding these ethical considerations will help you use AI responsibly.

9.3.1 AI Ethical Considerations

The discussion about the implications of AI in education and health care is ongoing and evolving (Shepherd & Griesheimer, 2024). However, one thing is clear: AI is here to stay. Given this reality, it's crucial to consider the ethical implications of AI use, particularly in nursing education.

A key ethical principle is that AI should be used to enhance work, not replace it (De Gagne

---

Table 9.1 AI skills and knowledge self-assessment

AI skills and knowledge statement	1	2	3	4	5
I understand what AI is and how it can be used in nursing education					
I am comfortable using AI tools like ChatGPT for learning support					
I use AI to clarify concepts I don't understand from my nursing lectures or readings					
I know how to formulate effective prompts to get useful information from AI					
I critically evaluate the information provided by AI before using it					
I use AI to generate practice questions or case studies when I prepare for exams					
I am aware of the ethical considerations about AI use in academic settings					
I can distinguish between appropriate and inappropriate uses of AI in my coursework					
I use AI to support my learning, not to replace my own critical thinking					
I am interested in learning more about how to effectively use AI in my nursing education.					

Total score:
1 = Strongly Disagree, 5 = Strongly Agree
Scoring:
    40–50: Advanced AI user
    30–39: Intermediate AI user
    20–29: Beginner AI user
    10–19: Novice AI user

et al., 2024). AI is a tool that requires a human partner to be truly effective and ethical. This is especially important in nursing, where critical thinking and human judgment are paramount.

When using AI as a learning tool in nursing school, it's critical to maintain academic integrity and avoid any form of cheating. The purpose of your nursing education is to develop the knowledge and skills you'll need to provide safe, competent patient care—not just to earn good grades. Using AI to complete assignments, write papers, or answer exam questions for you defeats that purpose and compromises your learning.

As a nursing student, you must preserve and develop your own critical thinking abilities rather than relying on AI to do the thinking for you. For example, if you're assigned to create a concept map about pressure wounds, using AI to generate the entire map for you bypasses the valuable learning process of applying your knowledge to link related concepts. The goal of such assignments is to engage your brain in ways that support retention and integration of nursing concepts.

It's also important to recognize that overreliance on AI could potentially compromise your nursing competence and ability to provide safe care in situations where AI isn't available. You need to develop and maintain your own knowledge and clinical reasoning skills. Additionally, be very cautious about inputting any patient information into AI tools, even if anonymized, to protect patient privacy and confidentiality.

While AI can be a powerful learning aid, it has limitations and can make mistakes or provide outdated information. As a nursing student and future nurse, you must develop the skills to critically evaluate information from any source. By keeping these ethical considerations in mind, you can harness AI's benefits to enhance your learning while maintaining the integrity of your education and future practice.

9.3.2 Examples of AI to Enhance Learning

In the examples that follow, you will see how a nursing student can use AI to enhance learning.

We will use one topic throughout the examples; tuberculosis. If you have not yet covered this topic in your nursing course you can still learn from these examples. Use your critical thinking to relate how you can apply these examples to any topic you are working to understand.

1. **Clarify a "Muddy Point"**

It is not uncommon in nursing schools to be introduced to topics in pre-reading or classes that even after the instructor reviews it, you still don't understand. In nursing education, we refer to that as a "muddy point," you may get the big picture about it but don't really understand the details.

Here's where we will begin our application using tuberculosis. You've had a class on transmission-based precautions and infectious diseases; tuberculosis was included. You did the readings and in class the instructor reviewed the two types of tuberculosis; Latent TB infection and Active TB disease. The instructor emphasized that airborne precautions are required for Active TB disease. You have used your critical thinking to conclude that there must be a difference between the two that is important based on this cue: Clients with Active TB disease need to be in airborne precautions, clients with Latent TB do not.

Don't use AI as a substitute for your own critical thinking. First attempt to solve this for yourself, and if you can't then turn to AI for help. You have already used your critical thinking to identify that there is an important difference. As you think about it more, you connect another cue; Active TB is contagious by respiratory secretions when the patient coughs or sneezes, and the bacteria that causes TB *Mycobacterium tuberculosis* is light enough that it hangs in the air. That would be why airborne precautions are required instead of droplet precautions. But you still can't explain why Latent TB does not require airborne precautions.

You will write your AI prompt. Here let's mention "prompt engineering." If you have used AI language models, you know that generating a response is different from doing a google search. Creating your prompt, or question to AI, and

9.3 AI in Nursing Education

revising it to refine the responses based on your need, is referred to as "prompt engineering."

You may need to work with prompts to get the answer you are looking for. Let's review some examples of prompts and the response you would get.

Example:

The following prompt: "In today's lecture about TB the instructor talked about Active TB and latent TB. I haven't heard of a communicable disease that had two different diseases like this. There must be an important difference that I don't get because we learned Active TB requires airborne precautions and Latent TB does not. Help me understand these two different types of the disease" gave this AI response.

Chat GPT Response:

"Active TB and latent TB are two different stages of the tuberculosis infection, which helps explain why they require different precautions and treatments.

- **Latent TB**: In latent TB, a person has been infected with the TB bacteria (*Mycobacterium tuberculosis*), but their immune system is able to keep it in check. The bacteria remain dormant in the body, and the person does not have symptoms, nor can they spread the disease to others. This is why no airborne precautions are necessary for latent TB. However, latent TB can reactivate, especially if the immune system becomes weakened, which is why treatment is often recommended to prevent progression to active TB.
- **Active TB**: In active TB, the bacteria overcome the immune system's defenses, causing symptoms such as coughing, weight loss, night sweats, and fever. Active TB is contagious, as the bacteria are present in the respiratory secretions and can be spread through the air when the infected person coughs, sneezes, or talks. This is why airborne precautions, such as the use of masks

and isolation rooms, are crucial for active TB to prevent transmission to others.

The distinction between latent and active TB is significant because it impacts both the treatment approach and the infection control measures needed. Latent TB is managed to prevent reactivation, while active TB requires treatment to cure the infection and prevent its spread."

Open AI (2024). *ChatGPT* (October 16 version) [Large language model]. https://chat.openai.com/chat

The response to your questions about the difference between Active and Latent TB is clear, but after reviewing it, you still don't feel like you can answer the "why" so you can write another prompt; "I need to understand WHY they are different." Remember, understanding "why" is one of the foundations of your critical thinking.

Again, you will write a prompt that clearly states what you are looking for. You will write "I see the difference between Active and Latent TB but I am still not clear on why there is a difference when it is the same disease, caused by a bacteria" and the following response:

ChatGPT response:
"1. Active TB:
   The immune system is unable to contain the bacteria effectively.
   The bacteria are actively multiplying and causing damage in the body, typically in the lungs.
   The person shows symptoms like coughing, fever, and weight loss.
   The person is contagious and can spread the bacteria to others.
2. Latent TB:
   - The immune system has successfully contained the bacteria.
   - The bacteria are present but dormant, like seeds that haven't sprouted.
   - The person shows no symptoms and feels healthy.

– The person is not contagious and cannot spread the bacteria.

The difference occurs because of variations in individual immune responses. A strong immune system can often contain TB bacteria, resulting in latent TB. However, if the immune system weakens (due to factors like stress, poor nutrition, or other illnesses), latent TB can activate.

Think of it like a fire:

– Active TB is like a burning fire, causing damage and able to spread.
– Latent TB is like embers under ashes—present but contained, with the potential to flare up if conditions change.

This distinction is crucial for treatment approaches and public health measures. Active TB requires immediate treatment and isolation precautions, while latent TB may be monitored or treated preventatively to stop potential activation."

Open AI (2024). *ChatGPT* (October 16 version) [Large language model]. https://chat.openai.com/chat ◄

Now you understand, and this understanding will help what you need to know about TB. This deeper understanding supports your brain-based learning and your critical thinking when you see case studies, clinical experiences, or test questions about tuberculosis.

2. **Create a Visual Learning Tool**

If you learn best when you have a picture or metaphor to help you understand a concept you use AI. You can ask for a visual image, like the one you got in the AI response to clarify a muddle point "Think of it like a fire." You can use that metaphor to draw your own image in your notes, and refer back to it as you study. Creating your own drawing based on the metaphor and including that in your study notes is an example of the brain-based learning strategy of interleaving.

You could use an AI image generator to create a concept map for you but as you do that, keep in mind this is not going to support your brain-based learning to the extent that your own work will.

3. **Apply a Case Study**

Another active learning strategy to support brain-based learning (Chap. 2) is using a case study to help link content to real-life scenarios. If you didn't get a case study in class, or in your textbook, you can create your own using AI.

Example:

Again, using TB, you can write this prompt "We learned about TB in class but didn't get a case study. Give me a TB case study."

ChatGPT response:
"Case Study: The Martinez Family TB Exposure

Background:
The Martinez family consists of Maria (32, mother), Carlos (35, father), Elena (10, daughter), and Luis (6, son). They recently immigrated to the United States from a country with a high TB prevalence.

Scenario:
During a routine health screening for her new job as a caregiver, Maria tests positive on a TB skin test. She is referred to the local health department for further evaluation.

Assessment:
1. Chest X-ray: Shows small cavitary lesions in the upper lobe of Maria's right lung.
2. Sputum test: Positive for *Mycobacterium tuberculosis*.
3. Symptoms: Maria reports a persistent cough for the past month, occasional night sweats, and recent weight loss.

Diagnosis:

Maria is diagnosed with active pulmonary tuberculosis.

Management:

1. Maria is started on a four-drug regimen: Isoniazid, Rifampin, Ethambutol, and Pyrazinamide.
2. She is placed on home isolation for the first 2 weeks of treatment.
3. A public health nurse is assigned to ensure treatment adherence through Directly Observed Therapy (DOT).

Family Screening:

1. Carlos, Elena, and Luis undergo TB screening.
2. Carlos and Elena have positive TB skin tests but normal chest X-rays and no symptoms.
3. Luis has a negative TB skin test.

Family Management:

1. Carlos and Elena are diagnosed with latent TB infection and offered preventive therapy.
2. Luis is scheduled for a follow-up TB test in 8–10 weeks due to possible recent exposure.
3. The family receives education on TB transmission, symptoms, and the importance of completing treatment.

Follow-up:

1. After 2 months, Maria's sputum tests negative for TB bacteria. She continues treatment for four more months.
2. Carlos and Elena complete their preventive therapy without complications.
3. Luis's follow-up test remains negative.

Learning Points:

1. Differentiate between active and latent TB infection.
2. Understand the importance of contact tracing in TB control.

3. Recognize the role of public health in managing TB cases.
4. Appreciate the significance of treatment adherence in TB management.
5. Identify the special considerations for TB in immigrant populations.

This case study provides a comprehensive overview of TB management, including diagnosis, treatment, public health measures, and family considerations."

Open AI (2024). *ChatGPT* (October 15 version) [Large language model]. ◄

The case study may help connect the concepts and support your learning. You may even think about the Martinez family and apply this case study to an exam question or a clinical scenario.

4. **Prepare for an Exam**

AI can be used cautiously to support your exam preparation. If you don't have access to a test bank with practice questions, you can use AI to create them. You would not want to use this as your only resource for exam question review, because the AI will not know what your instructor will emphasize on the exam. In addition, the exam questions you generate would be for your review, not for sharing with other students.

Example:

Let's mention again the importance of prompt engineering. You will need to let your AI know that you are a nursing student, and what level courses you are taking. Here's a sample prompt:

> I want to review for my exam in my next nursing class. I'm a nursing student in my first clinical course and TB is a topic on the exam. The instructor talked about active TB, latent TB, care of the TB client using airborne precautions, TB medication regimens, and also mentioned TB testing and BCG vaccine. Give me 5 exam questions with rationale for the correct answer at the end so I can take the questions before seeing the answers.

ChatGPT response:

"1. A client with latent TB asks you why they need to take medication when they feel perfectly healthy. What is the most appropriate response?

   (A) 'Taking the medication will prevent you from developing active TB'.

   (B) 'The medication is given to relieve your symptoms'.

   (C) 'You're required to take it as part of hospital policy'.

   (D) 'It's just a precaution, and you can stop taking it whenever you want'.

2. Which medication regimen is commonly used to treat active TB due to its effectiveness and ability to prevent drug resistance?

   (A) Rifampin (RIF), Isoniazid (INH), Ethambutol (EMB), Pyrazinamide (PZA)

   (B) Isoniazid (INH) alone

   (C) Ethambutol (EMB) and Streptomycin (SM)

   (D) Rifampin (RIF) and Pyrazinamide (PZA)

3. What is the primary reason for administering a Tuberculin Skin Test (TST) or a TB blood test (IGRA)?

   (A) To confirm the presence of active TB

   (B) To differentiate between active and latent TB

   (C) To monitor the effectiveness of TB treatment

   (D) To assess the client's immunity to TB

4. The nurse is caring for a client with active TB in an airborne isolation room. The client is experiencing increased coughing and is producing sputum. What should the nurse do first?

   (A) Ensure that the negative pressure in the room is functioning properly.

   (B) Administer a prescribed cough suppressant medication.

   (C) Provide the client with a tissue to cover their mouth and nose when coughing.

   (D) Leave the room and inform the charge nurse of the client's condition.

5. Why is the BCG vaccine not routinely administered in the United States?

   (A) The vaccine is not effective in preventing TB.

   (B) The vaccine may cause severe adverse reactions.

   (C) The vaccine interferes with TB testing results.

   (D) The vaccine is too expensive for widespread use.

1. A

   Taking the medication will prevent you from developing active TB. Treatment of Latent TB is for the purpose of preventing future progression of Latent TB infection to active TB disease.

2. A

   The combination of Rifampin (RIF), Isoniazid (INH), Ethambutol (EMB), and Pyrazinamide (PZA) is the standard regimen for treating active TB.

3. B

   Tuberculin Skin Tests (TST) or TB blood tests are used to detect the presence of TB antigen which indicates to the mycobacterium bacillus.

4. C

   Clients should be reminded to cover their mouth and nose when they cough or sneeze to prevent the spread of the bacillus into the air.

5. C

   The BCG vaccine can interfere with TB testing results, making it less useful for diagnostic purposes."

Open AI (2024). *ChatGPT* (January 28 version) [Large language model]. ◄

You can use sample exam questions like this to support your brain-based learning and critical thinking. Now you have an opportunity to learn more about this topic, which will help you prepare for exams. The most important aspect of your learning when you create and review exam questions is to support your understanding of the topic, in this case, TB. Of course, you would not see these same questions on an exam, but review of the questions helps you to learn and understand the content.

These examples related to a student learning about TB are just a few of the unlimited ways you can use AI to enhance your brain-based learning and critical thinking in nursing school. If you've not used AI, you'll want to experiment with different prompts and remember that **AI is not always accurate**. You will need to use your critical thinking when you review AI responses. If something doesn't seem right, it's probably not. Explore further, ask more questions, and in the end, trust yourself.

5. Navigate the Complexity of Nursing School

We have already agreed that nursing school is difficult. Keeping focused on a growth and learning mindset over a performance mindset can be a burden, especially when you have not performed well. Even though AI is not sentient (it does not have feelings) it can give you feedback if you are struggling.

Example:

If you're feeling overwhelmed at a point in time, try reaching out to AI for advice. Let's be clear, AI does not replace mental health support, but might be able to give you tips on learning strategy. For example, a prompt like this: "I am really discouraged. I studied hard for my last exam, reviewed content on TB and even took practice questions. I missed three of the five questions about TB and I'm at risk for not passing the course" generates the following response.

ChatGPT response:
"I understand you're feeling discouraged. It's normal to feel this way after putting in effort and not seeing the results you hoped for. However, this setback doesn't define your abilities or your future as a nursing student. Let's look at this situation constructively:

1. Analyze your performance:
   - Review the questions you missed. Were they about specific details, or did they require applying knowledge to scenarios?
   - Identify any patterns in the types of questions you struggled with.
2. Adjust your study strategy:
   - Consider using more active learning techniques like creating concept maps or teaching the material to someone else.
   - Focus on understanding the "why" behind concepts, not just memorizing facts.
3. Seek help:
   - Talk to your instructor about the areas you're struggling with. They may offer insights or additional resources.
   - Consider forming a study group or finding a tutor who can explain concepts in a different way.
4. Practice application:
   - Find or create more practice questions that focus on applying TB knowledge to patient scenarios.
   - Review case studies to better understand how TB knowledge is used in real-world situations.
5. Manage stress:
   - Ensure you're getting enough sleep and taking care of your physical health.
   - Practice stress-reduction techniques like deep breathing or mindfulness.
6. Keep perspective:
   - Remember that learning is a process. It's okay to struggle with difficult concepts at first.
   - Focus on progress rather than perfection. How has your understanding improved since you started studying TB?

7. Plan your next steps:
   - Break down the remaining course content into manageable chunks.
   - Create a study schedule that allows for regular review of challenging topics.

Remember, many successful nurses have faced similar challenges during their education. Your dedication to improving shows that you have the persistence needed to succeed in nursing. Don't give up—you can overcome this obstacle and become the nurse you aspire to be."

Open AI (2024). *ChatGPT* (October 13 version) [Large language model]. ◀

So you see, not only did the AI provide word of support, but also gave practical advice.

These are examples using ChatGPT. As noted earlier in the chapter, there are other AI tools you can use. The more you work with an AI tool the better you will become at learning how to use prompts to guide you.

9.3.3   AI Do's and Don'ts

As you can see from the examples, AI is useful for augmenting your learning and even for giving you tips for success, many of which look familiar to the content in this book! Table 9.2 outlines things to keep in mind when using AI.

The bottom link is that you should in all circumstances use AI with a growth mindset for learning, not with a fixed mindset for completing tasks. Table 9.3 contrasts using a growth mindset and using a fixed mindset when relying on AI.

By incorporating AI responsibly, you can enhance your learning experience and develop critical thinking skills that are essential for success in nursing school and beyond. From clarifying complex concepts to generating practice scenarios, AI can be a powerful tool in your learning journey. It is crucial to remember AI is

Table 9.2 AI do's and don'ts

Do	Don't
Use AI for additional information on topics you are learning	Take shortcuts or use AI to complete assignments
Refine your prompt engineering to get responses just for you	Generate references for written assignments. AI tools in general do not have access to all databases and may generate a reference that looks legitimate but does not exist
Review AI responses using your critical thinking; AI is not perfect and can make things up	Rely solely on AI for exam preparation or for learning assignments
Set up an account and be consistent with using it. The AI will "learn" how to respond to your learning needs and tailor responses accordingly.	Share your AI account or prompts with others. Your account will become personalized to you and sharing it with others will compromise the personalization of your responses

Table 9.3 Growth mindset and fixed mindset use of AI

Growth mindset with AI	Fixed mindset with AI
Think it through yourself *before* asking AI. Your brain-based learning is enhanced when you figure it out for yourself	Using AI for cheating, in any way, shape or form. AI should not replace your thinking
Ask AI to confirm your thinking. If you have worked it out for yourself, you can ask AI if you got it right	Use AI to complete an assignment instead of writing it yourself
Ask AI to add to your learning; write a case study, create practice questions, create a jeopardy game	Use AI for references; they may be "generated" and not actual publications and can be inaccurate
Critically evaluate AI responses	Use AI to search for quizzes or tests that have already been given. Most AI applications have "guardrails" that will prohibit the duplication of a test or exam that is found on the internet

meant to augment, not replace, your critical thinking and problem-solving skills. It is your responsibility to use it ethically.

9.3.4 AI and the Future in Nursing Education and Practice

The landscape of AI in health care and nursing education is evolving at an unprecedented pace. By the time you read this, many of the "future trends" discussed here will be in use! This rapid evolution underscores the importance of maintaining an open mind and staying informed about the latest developments in AI.

The future of AI in nursing education holds exciting possibilities. We may soon see highly personalized learning experiences, with AI tailoring content and teaching methods to individual student needs and learning styles. This could revolutionize how you learn and apply nursing knowledge.

In clinical training, AI-enhanced virtual and augmented reality simulations are set to provide increasingly realistic scenarios. These advanced simulations will allow you to practice critical skills and decision making in a safe, controlled environment that is more flexible than your simulation lab experiences.

As you progress in your nursing career, you're likely to encounter more sophisticated AI tools designed to support clinical decision making. These systems may assist in patient assessment, care planning, and even predictive analytics for patient outcomes. As with all AI, these tools will complement rather than replace human clinical judgment.

With these expansions will come a continued emphasis on ethical use of AI and you will have a commitment to holding the highest standard of ethics as you use AI in your nursing education and practice.

AI is a powerful tool but it does not replace the human skills—empathy, critical thinking, and clinical judgment—that will define you as an outstanding nurse. Use AI to enhance these skills, not replace them.

9.4 Conclusion

AI offers powerful tools to enhance your nursing education, from clarifying complex concepts to generating practice scenarios. Use AI as a supplement to, not a replacement for, your critical thinking skills. By maintaining a growth mindset and using AI responsibly, you can deepen your understanding of nursing concepts, prepare effectively for exams, and navigate nursing school challenges with confidence. As you integrate AI into your studies, always prioritize ethical use and balance technological assistance with the irreplaceable human skills at the core of nursing practice.

Part II of this book has equipped you with essential tools for nursing school success that enhance your ability to apply critical thinking as you learn to think like a nurse. These skills are crucial for your journey through nursing education and into your professional career. In Part III, we will explore considerations for your first nursing job that will provide you with valuable insights even if you're just beginning your nursing education. We'll then delve into the NCLEX exam so that you understand the basics of the structure of the NCLEX and why committing to building your foundation of knowledge throughout nursing school is essential. The remainder of Part III will provide you with valuable NCLEX preparation resources that will lead you to NCLEX success.

Chapter 9 Synthesis Learning Activity: Applying AI with a Growth Mindset

After exploring the examples of using AI in nursing education you can apply your learning from this chapter. Consider a challenging concept from one of your recent nursing courses. Then, complete the following exercise:

1. Identify the challenging topic you've recently covered in one of your nursing courses.
2. Describe how you could use AI with a growth mindset to enhance your understanding of this concept.

References

Alowais, S. A., Alghamdi, S. S., Alsuhebany, N., Alqahtani, T., Alshaya, A. I., Almohareb, S. N., et al. (2023). Revolutionizing healthcare: The role of artificial intelligence in clinical practice. *BMC Medical Education, 23*(1), 689.

Bumbach, M. D. (2024). The use of AI powered ChatGPT for nursing education. *Journal of Nursing Education, 63*(8), 564–567. https://doi.org/10.3928/01484834-20240318-04

De Gagne, J. C., Hwang, H., & Jung, D. (2024). Cyberethics in nursing education: Ethical implications of artificial intelligence. *Nursing Ethics, 31*(6), 1021–1030. https://doi.org/10.1177/09697330231201901

Douthit, B., Shaw, R. D., Lytle, K. S., Richesson, R. L., & Cary, M. P., (2022, January 11). Artificial intelligence in nursing. *American Nurse.* https://www.myamericannurse.com/ai-artificial-intelligence-in-nursing/

Foronda, C. L., Gonzalez, L., Meese, M. M., Slamon, N., Baluyot, M., Lee, J., & Aebersold, M. (2024). A comparison of virtual reality to traditional simulation in health professions education: A systematic review. *Simulation in Healthcare.* https://doi.org/10.1097/SIH.0000000000000745

Shepherd, J., & Griesheimer, D. (2024). FAQs: AI and prompt engineering: The future of nursing education and professional development. *American Nurse Journal, 19*(6), 14–19. https://doi.org/10.51256/anj062414

Simms, R. C. (2025). Generative artificial intelligence (AI) literacy in nursing education: A crucial call to action. *Nurse Education Today, 146,* 106544.

Part III

NCLEX and Career Planning

Finding Your Ideal First Nursing Job

10

Your first job is the beginning of a journey, not the destination.

—Unknown

10.1 Introduction

As you progress through your nursing program, it's helpful to start thinking ahead about your first job as a nurse. Finding the right position to begin your nursing career is an exciting but sometimes overwhelming process. This chapter will guide you through important considerations about your first nursing job. This knowledge will also help you make the most of your experience during nursing school. We'll explore key factors like transition-to-practice programs, organizational culture, and unit environments that can significantly impact your early career experience. By understanding what to look for and how to approach your job search, you'll be better prepared to find a position that sets you up for long-term success in nursing.

▶ **By the end of this chapter you will be able to:**
1. Describe the nursing job market for new graduates and how it impacts a job search.
2. Compare and contrast different clinical areas for new graduate nurses (e.g., med/surg, critical care, ED).
3. Identify key elements of effective nurse residency and transition-to-practice programs.
4. Evaluate organizational culture and unit-level factors that contribute to positive work environments for new nurses.
5. Develop a strategic plan for a nursing job search.

10.2 Your Nursing Future: From Student to Professional Nurse

It's common for nursing students to think about their first nursing job long before applying for jobs in their final semester. Many students enter nursing school with a clear vision of where they want to work—perhaps inspired by personal experiences, media portrayals of nursing, or a particular health issue they're passionate about.

It is important to keep an open mind as you progress through your program. You can be surprised to find your interests shift as you gain exposure to different areas of nursing. Each clini-

© The Author(s), under exclusive license to Springer Nature Switzerland AG 2025
C. Thompson, *Nursing School, NCLEX and Career Transition Success*,
https://doi.org/10.1007/978-3-031-85538-2_10

cal rotation, each class, and each interaction with health care professionals provides an opportunity to learn not just about nursing care, but about yourself as a future nurse. Pay attention to what excites you, what challenges you, and what type of environment makes you feel most energized and fulfilled.

You will act on the decisions about where you begin your nursing career by applying for, interviewing, and accepting a job before you finish nursing school. Most students do this in their final semester of nursing school.

Many nursing students work in a hospital or while they are in school or as a nurse extern during a semester break and plan to continue at that hospital to work as an RN. In some cases, they may even have a position offer as part of a tuition loan forgiveness or sign on commitment.

You may have an idea where you want to apply to begin your nursing career, and you may even be taking on the start of your nursing career as an opportunity to grab an adventure with a relocation to a new city or state. Either way there are some things you should consider.

10.2.1 The Nursing Shortage

You already know there is a shortage of RNs in the United States. Projections from the Bureau of Labor Statistics indicate that the job market for registered nurses is growing faster than average. Over the next decade, it's expected that there will be nearly 200,000 openings for RNs each year. This growth reflects the continuing high demand for nursing professionals across the country (US Bureau of Labor Statistics, 2024).

Go to any hospital website under nursing positions and you will see many RN[1] opportunities. However, there are limited openings for new graduate nurses. This is because orienting a new

graduate nurse is expensive and time consuming for a health care organization. If you are in a diploma or associate degree program, you may not be offered a position before a bachelor's applicant. This is because when you are hired for an RN position without a bachelor's degree, the health care organization is going to have to invest in your continuing education for you to pursue that degree.

Because there is a shortage of nurses, hospitals are desperate to fill RN positions and may offer hefty incentives like sign on bonuses to entice you. Be cautious of beginning your first nursing position in a hospital that is desperate for nurses. The likelihood of becoming dissatisfied with your career is far greater when you don't get a solid transition with support. Limit your job search to hospitals that support new nurses in their transition to nursing.

10.2.2 Planning Your Nursing Job

Unless you are working during school in the health care organization where you have been guaranteed an RN position you will need to apply and interview for a position. If you have not already given thought to where you would want to work as a nurse, get serious about planning your options BEFORE your final year of nursing school. This is particularly important if you are graduating from your program in May, when new graduate positions are more competitive.

If your nursing school curriculum does not include a course that integrates job search content you will have to navigate this process on your own. If you have a Nursing Leadership or similar course in your final semester that supports your job search, you may need to begin some of your job search activity before that course starts.

If you are working in a hospital in any role, it is not safe to assume you will automatically get a new nurse position when you graduate. Just like other students who are going through the job search process, you'll want to reach out to the

---

[1] As noted in the book Introduction, the resources support students in practical nurse (PN) programs as well as students in RN programs. In this chapter the focus is on RN positions. If you are in a PN school of nursing, your nursing school should have career resources available for you.

10.2 Your Nursing Future: From Student to Professional Nurse

department that hires nurses and make sure you understand their process for transitioning to a new nurse position.

10.2.3 Starting as a GN or Waiting to Pass NCLEX

In some states, you cannot begin your position as a new nurse until you have passed NCLEX and are a licensed RN. You can still begin your job search and secure a position.

In some states, you can obtain a temporary practice permit and begin work as a Graduate Nurse (GN) then transition to an RN position after you pass NCLEX. If you intend to apply in a state where you can work as a GN, Table 10.1 outlines things to consider.

Starting directly as an RN after passing NCLEX has its own set of advantages and challenges. On the positive side, you'll have the ability to focus entirely on NCLEX preparation without the added stress of work responsibilities. This dedicated study time can be invaluable, allowing you to approach the exam with your full attention and energy.

Additionally, beginning your career with your RN license in hand can provide a sense of confidence. You won't have to navigate the transition from GN to RN status, which can be stressful.

Many health care organizations will have a set time frame within which you must pass NCLEX to secure or maintain your job offer. This can create added stress as you complete your postgraduation NCLEX preparation.

10.2.4 Choosing Your First Nursing Position

Whether you're just starting nursing school or nearing graduation, it's never too early (or too late) to start thinking about where you want your nursing career to begin. If you are early in your nursing program, this information will guide your choices about clinical experiences (if you have an option to select them), extracurricular activities, and work choices. If you are nearing graduation you will be taking actionable steps outlined in this section.

Where you begin your nursing career is just that—a beginning. It's important to remember that your first job is not a lifelong commitment, but rather a stepping stone in your professional journey. Many nurses change specialties or work settings several times throughout their careers, each move bringing new learning opportunities and professional growth.

Your initial choice of nursing environment can significantly impact your early career experiences, skill development, and future opportunities. Different settings offer varying levels of acuity, client populations, and learning curves. Some may align more closely with your current interests or long-term goals, while others might challenge you in unexpected ways.

In this section, we'll explore common hospital settings where new graduate nurses begin their careers. The advantages and potential challenges of each are presented to help you to make an informed decision about what is best for you.

Table 10.1 Advantages and disadvantages of starting as a GN

Advantages of starting as a GN	Disadvantages of starting as a GN
Hourly wage closer to RN salary	Limited time for NCLEX prep with full time work schedule
Opportunity to earn income sooner	Potential for increased stress balancing work and NCLEX prep
May allow paid time off for NCLEX prep	If the first NCLEX attempt is not successful can have significant consequences such as demotion, pay cut, or retraction of RN position
May offer classes for NCLEX prep	Potential for role confusion when transitioning from GN to RN role
Clinical experience supports application of learning for NCLEX prep	Less flexibility in scheduling NCLEX test date due to work schedule

There's no universally "best" option—the right choice depends on your individual skills, interests, and career aspirations.

10.2.5 Starting in Med/Surg

Starting on a med/surg unit is a common choice for many nursing school graduates. Advantages and disadvantages of this choice are outlined on Table 10.2.

For students who aspire to begin in a specialty unit, things to consider are outlined in Table 10.3.

Emergency Department (ED) nursing is complex, and many hospitals do not hire new graduates to begin in the Emergency Department. However, it can be a popular option for nursing students who believe they will be energized by the fast paced adrenaline rush that can happen in a busy ED. Things to consider are outlined in Table 10.4.

Just like with Emergency Department nursing, many hospitals do not hire new graduates to begin in the specialty units like Labor, Delivery. Postpartum, Pediatric or Mental Health. It will be easier for you to move in the future from med/surg to a unit like this than it would be to move from this speciality care setting to another setting.

Table 10.2 Beginning in med/surg

Beginning in med/surg	
Advantages	Disadvantages
Exposure to a variety of diagnosis	High patient load can be overwhelming
Build foundational nursing skills; assessment, medication administration, wound care, discharge planning, patient education	Less opportunity for in-depth focus on specific conditions or treatments
Develop time management and organizational skills	Potentially higher stress levels due to diverse patient needs
Good foundational preparation for future specialization	Less time for extended patient relationships due to shorter stays

Table 10.3 Beginning in critical care

Beginning in acute care specialty unit	
Advantages	Disadvantages
Caring for high acuity patients with complex medical needs can be intellectually challenging and rewarding	Steep learning curve; nursing practice in a critical care typically builds on foundational knowledge that a novice nurse would not possess
Opportunity to develop specialized knowledge	Limited patient diversity depending on the unit
Work with advanced technology	Emotional toll of helplessness and grief when patients do not recover
Fast paced	Higher risk for career "burnout"

Table 10.4 Beginning in ED

Beginning in the emergency department	
Advantages	Disadvantages
Variety of clinical cases and diagnoses offer opportunity for expansive learning	Steep learning curve; nursing practice in a emergency department typically builds on foundational knowledge that a novice nurse would not possess
Fast paced environment to develop strong assessment, prioritization and clinical decision making skills	Greater risk for workplace violence from patients and visitors
Satisfaction in seeing immediate impact of interventions	Emotional toll of helplessness and grief when patients do not recover
Fast paced	Limited opportunity to develop relationships with clients

10.2.6 Where You Begin Is Just Your Beginning

You have a long and exciting career ahead of you. Nursing provides unlimited opportunities for growth in a wide variety of areas. You can move into advanced clinical practice by pursuing further education to become a Nurse Practitioner, Nurse Midwife, or Nurse Anesthetist. You can do travel nursing. You can move into a leadership role. You could transition to a setting like the ones listed above, or another such as anesthesia care either in the OR or postanesthesia recovery (PACU), in radiology, in infusion, or in the cardiac cath lab.

You could pursue a practice setting outside of the hospital such as hospital at home, home health nursing, ambulatory care nursing, home infusion, or a virtual nurse role. You could become a school nurse, work in public health or in occupational health. You could even become a legal nurse consultant. You have so many opportunities.

Keep this in mind as you ponder this decision about where you will begin your nursing career. You are not making a lifelong commitment to a particular hospital or setting, but should try to give yourself at least 2 years in the place where you start to develop your clinical decision making skills that you can then apply when you move into your next role.

You are launching what should be a long and exciting career. Your important task now is to set your course for your short-term goal; successful transition to your nursing career. This sets the stage for you to accomplish great things in your nursing future.

10.3 📝 Practical Strategies: Preparing for Your Job Search

These practical strategies will get you started on your job search process.

- **Set your vision**

This is an important time to revisit why you decided to go to nursing school. In the midst of all your hard work, maybe you lost track of why you wanted to be a nurse.

For your job search, you'll want to keep your long-term vision in mind while also considering that for the short term, your goal is to make a successful transition to nursing practice. Employers who will be hiring you as a graduate nurse are investing in supporting this transition.

When you write your resume and prepare for your job interviews you will need to be able to define your vision for your nursing career and what sets you apart from other new graduate nurses. When you write your vision statement, be clear that you are embarking on your nursing career as a new graduate nurse, eager to begin your journey to becoming an expert nurse clinician.

As a new graduate nurse, you are somewhat of a liability; the hospital that hires you will be investing a great deal into your transition-to-practice. You will not be functioning independently for 6–12 months. They are not going to be enticed to hire you if your vision is to use your first position as a stepping stone to going back to school or transferring to another setting after 1 year.

If you are a traditional student and your clinical experience has been limited to what you had in nursing school your vision statement may be:

> As a new nursing graduate, my vision is to journey from novice nurse within the framework of a Nurse Residency program to launch my nursing career and fulfill my lifelong dream of being a nurse. I am committed to applying my foundational nursing education to become the best nurse I can be.

If you are a traditional student with a life experience that shaped your desire to be a nurse your vision statement may be:

> My desire to become a nurse was rooted in my experience as a childhood cancer survivor, and now look forward to embarking on my journey to embody the best of what I experienced as a child.

If you are a traditional student with health care-related clinical experience outside of your nursing school clinical you don't want to oversell that experience; being a nursing assistant is not the same as being a nurse. Your vision statement may be:

> As a new nursing graduate, my vision is to launch my nursing career and fulfill my lifelong dream of being a nurse. My previous health care clinical

experience has provided valuable skills that I recognize does not replace nursing practice experience but has honed my awareness of the passion I have for nursing.

If you are a second degree student with previous work experience you may link that to your vision statement such as:

My desire to become a nurse stemmed from my previous experience as a laboratory technician, where I witnessed the impact nurses have on their patients. I now seek to embark on my journey to fulfilling my dream of becoming a nurse within the framework that will support my transition to practice.

- **Draft your resume**

Your college, university, or school of nursing should have a Career Placement or Career Advising office where you can get assistance with writing your resume.

You can also find resume resources and templates online. Your resume should include:

1. Your name, address and contact information.
2. A SHORT Vision Statement (see #1 above).
3. Overview of sites where you have had clinical experience.
4. Nursing conferences you have attended.
5. Awards you have received.
6. Health care work experience.
7. Non-health-care work experience to demonstrate your work ethics.

You may want to fine tune your resume based on a particular job you decide to pursue. You may also find that a health care organization has an application process that will not require a resume as part of the application process. However, the process of writing your resume helps organize your experience and will prepare you to highlight your vision and attributes when you interview for a position.

You can use AI using examples described in Chap. 9 to improve your resume, but don't use it to write your resume. A resume that looks like it was written by AI will create a red flag.

- **Attend job fairs**

Even if you think you know where you want to work after graduation, if your school of nursing has a job fair, attend it. You might find an opportunity that entices you more than what you had been considering and you will get experience presenting yourself in an interview environment.

Guidelines for attending a job fair:

- Prepare in advance.
  - Research the organizations represented and list the ones you want to speak with.
- Bring your resume.
  - Carrying paper copies of your resume in a professional and organized way.
- Dress professionally.
  - A contact at a Job Fair is the same as an interview. Dress the part.
- Go on your own.
  - Don't travel through the Job Fair with a pack of friends. You want to focus on the representatives from hospitals who are hiring graduate nurses and sell yourself.

- **Network and join professional organizations**

Networking and involvement in professional organizations can significantly enhance your job search and career prospects. You might want to join your school's Student Nurses' Association or local chapter of the National Student Nurses' Association (NSNA). These organizations often host career events and provide job search resources.

You could also consider becoming a student member of professional nursing organizations related to your interests, such as the American Nurses Association (ANA) or specialty-specific organizations like the Emergency Nurses Association (ENA) or the American Association of Critical-Care Nurses (AACN).

You can use social media platforms like LinkedIn to connect with nurses and health care professionals in your area of interest.

10.3 Practical Strategies: Preparing for Your Job Search

Networking can help you learn about job openings before they're publicly posted, gain insider knowledge about different health care organizations, and secure recommendations.

- **Consider who will be your references**

Most applications will ask you to provide references. In most cases you will not be asked to provide reference letters but instead will provide reference contact information. Individuals who are your references will then receive an online form to complete.

You should select references who know you and can speak to your abilities as a future nurse; a course or clinical instructors, an adviser in your nursing program, a mentor in a clinical rotation, or a supervisor in your work if you work in a health care setting while you are in nursing school.

When you are ready to complete an application and list a reference, be sure to speak to that individual BEFORE you give their name and contact information. This is a professional courtesy that you do not want to overlook.

- **Plan ahead so you're not left behind**

Hospitals that are nurse-friendly places where nurses want to work will have a new graduate transition program with a limited number of spaces. You don't want to miss out on your best first opportunity by waiting too long to begin looking.

Begin with a list of hospitals where you think you'd like to work. Check their websites for application timelines and reach out to their nurse recruiters.

Even though your senior year, and in particular your final semester in school is busy, you will want to plan ahead so that you can make time for interviews.

Because hospitals start new graduate hires in structured orientation programs, if you wait until after your graduation to begin looking for a job, you may wait until the next new graduate hiring sequence to begin your job. Complete the Pause

and Reflect 10.1 to begin working on drafting your vision.

▶ **Pause and Reflect 10.1: Setting Your Vision** Take a moment to reflect on your decision to pursue nursing as a career and your vision for your nursing career.

If you're early in your program, consider how your vision might evolve as you gain more clinical experience. Write what your vision statement would have been before you started and compare that to a vision statement you would write now. If you're near graduation, reflect on how your vision has changed since you started nursing school. Write the vision statement you will include on your resume.

No matter where you are in your nursing program, it is never too early to think about your resume. Complete Pause and Reflect 10.2 to begin a draft of your resume.

▶ **Pause and Reflect 10.2: Draft Your Resume** If you are early in your nursing program, focus on what you hope to include on your resume by the time you graduate. What aspects of your education do you want to highlight? What could you plan to fill gaps in your experience before you graduate? How does your resume align with your vision statement? What strategies will you need to consider so that you can achieve your goals for what to have accomplished before you graduate?

If you are near graduation, use this pause and reflect to draft your actual resume. Focus on how you present your nursing education and experience.

10.3.1 Begin Your Search: What to Consider for Your First Position

As you conduct your search keep in mind three key factors that will help ensure a smoother transition into nursing practice: the organization's transition-to-practice support for new graduates, the organization's culture that supports nursing, and the unit culture that supports nurse satisfaction. Each of these are pivotal to your satisfaction in your first nursing position.

- **Nurse Residency or structured transition to practice for new graduate nurses**

Your first year transition to nursing practice is a big adventure. Nursing school has taught you what you need to get started, but you will be starting as a novice nurse. In her influential work on the topic of competence in practice, Dr. Patricia Benner (1982) identified that nurses move through five stages of development: novice, advanced beginner, competent, proficient, and expert.

No matter how much experience you have had in clinical as a nursing student, or in a job as an extern or nursing assistant, you will begin as a novice nurse. In your first months of practice, you will transition from novice to advanced beginner. While every nurse progresses at their own pace, with structured support most nurses can progress to competent practice within their first year. This is why many hospitals offer Nurse Residency programs for new graduate hires that are often up to 12 months long. These programs recognize that the journey from novice to competent practice requires structured support and guidance throughout the first year.

Coordinated and lengthy transition-to-practice programs, like a nurse residency program (NRP), are an evidence-based intervention for improving the likelihood that a new nurse will be satisfied as they progress through the transition to nursing (Goode et al., 2018; Knighten, 2022). In addition, NRPs have been linked to improved client outcomes when a new nurse is responsible for client care (Webb et al., 2024).

Given the support an NRP offers new graduates to support their transition to practice, you may want to prioritize that in your job search. If a hospital offers a big salary, or sign on bonus that is enticing, be sure to also consider what they have in place to support your transition to practice. If instead of a structured NRP they offer a loosely defined "shadowing" or orientation phase

you may want to think twice about beginning your nursing career there.

- **Organizational culture that supports nursing**

Organizational culture has a strong influence on job satisfaction for all of their workers, nurses included (Cunningham et al., 2024). An organization that has poor leadership, poor communication, limited resources, and chronic understaffing is not an ideal setting for you to begin your career.

You know from meeting nurses and working on various units in your clinical experiences that not all nurses are happy nurses, and not all units are happy places to work. In general, an organizational culture impacts interpersonal relationships within and among units (Banaszak-Holl et al., 2015) and therefore when you see a healthy and employee-centered organizational culture you are likely to see a nursing organizational culture that will support your career transition.

ANA Magnet Recognition ANA Magnet or Pathway Designation will be noted on the hospital's website and reflects not just that the hospital has a Nurse Residency program, but also that the hospital has an organizational culture that supports nursing practice.

If a hospital you are considering has ANA Magnet or Pathway Designation then you know they have met rigorous criteria that aligns with organizational culture that supports nursing. You can also explore other information about the hospital or health care system such as quality, client satisfaction, and employee satisfaction data.

Quality Ratings or Designations There are numerous quality indicators that reflect organizational performance. Health care organizations are required to report hospital data about patient outcomes. These data are compiled and used for various rankings. Medicare ranks by number of stars; one to five; with five star rating being the highest. Leapfrog is another agency that ranks quality and safety outcomes data. These are just two examples of sources of data. There are many other designations of quality and those would be listed on the hospital or health care organization website.

Client Satisfaction Data Hospitals and health care systems are required to collect and report client satisfaction data, referred to as the Hospital Consumer Assessment of Healthcare Providers and Systems, or HCAHPS data. Because the relationship between nurse satisfaction and client outcomes has been well documented, these HCAHPS data also give you information about the nursing environment. If the system has high client satisfaction scores, you can be more confident it is a place you would want to work. These scores are easily viewed at a website called Hospital Compare.

Employee Satisfaction Information Some hospitals and health care organizations publish employee satisfaction data. "Best Places to Work" rankings are publicly available. If an employer has been recognized as having distinction in employee satisfaction they are likely to note that on their website.

These are all attributes for you to consider as you gather information about nursing culture.

- **Unit culture that supports nurse satisfaction**

When deciding on a nursing position, it's essential to interview not just the organization but also the specific unit. Even in an organization that has a supportive nursing culture, you can find a nursing unit that is not cohesive. A unit culture is just as important as the organizational culture in supporting nurse well-being and job satisfaction (Leep & Stimpfel, 2024).

If you have experience working or in a unit, you benefit from understanding its culture. On the other hand, if you are pursuing a position in a hospital and in a unit that is new to you, as part of your search, you will want to gather information about the unit. After your hard work making it through nursing school, you do not want to start your career in a setting where that will stifle and frustrate you.

During interviews, speak with the unit clinical manager and several nurses to understand the unit's dynamics. Inquire about unit turnover rates, as high turnover can indicate a problematic culture that may not support well-being. Avoid accepting a position without thoroughly "interviewing" the unit, as this will be your professional home during a critical career phase. Ensure the unit culture aligns with your needs for a positive and supportive transition into nursing practice.

The following is a list of questions you could consider asking to learn more about unit culture:

- Do employees have opportunities for recognition?
- Is there a structured mentorship program?
- Are there regular team meetings?
- Is decision making collaborative?
- Are professional development opportunities available?
- Is work–life balance supported?
- Are there team social activities?
- Are communication channels clear?

Now that you understand more about factors associated with easing your transition to nursing practice, a structured orientation program as well as organizational and unit culture that supports nursing, consider these in relation to your vision for your first job. Complete Pause and Reflect 10.3.

Pause and Reflect 10.3: My Job Search Priorities

Reflect on and record your answer these questions:

1. What are your nonnegotiables for your first nursing position? List your top three must-haves and explain why each is essential to you.
2. What potential barriers might you face in your job search (location restrictions, schedule needs, etc.)? How might you address these?
3. What resources are available to help you with your search? List specific people, organizations, and tools you can utilize.

10.3.2 Prioritizing Your Job Search

Your final months in nursing school are busy, which risks making your job search take a back seat in that hectic schedule. However, securing your ideal first nursing job is an important step in launching your career. To ensure you don't miss out on opportunities, it's essential to prioritize this task.

Keep your eye on the goal and make time for the work. Allocate time for job search activities. This includes researching potential employers, preparing your resume, attending job fairs, and scheduling interviews. Treat these activities with the same importance as your academic responsibilities.

The effort you put into your job search will pay off significantly in the long run. A well-planned job search can lead to a position that offers a supportive environment, opportunities for growth, and a strong foundation for your nursing career. Making time for this process is an investment in your future success.

10.4 Conclusion

Finding your ideal first nursing job is an exciting and critical step in your nursing career. By understanding the job market, exploring different clinical settings, and considering factors like transition programs and organizational culture, you'll be well-equipped to make an informed decision. Remember, your first job is a stepping stone, not a final destination. Stay open to learning opportunities and remain focused on your long-term career goals.

While planning your first position is crucial, it goes hand in hand with ensuring your NCLEX success. After all, passing the NCLEX is your ticket to beginning your nursing career. The next two chapters will provide you with everything you need to know about the NCLEX, from application to examination. Consider it your comprehensive guide to this important milestone. Just as you've strategically approached your job search, you'll want to be strategic about your NCLEX success.

Chapter 10 Synthesis Learning Activity: My Job Search

The purpose of this assignment is to create a roadmap for your career transition from nursing student to nurse and assemble the information you will need for your initial job search. If you are a beginning nursing student, this will help you set a guide for your thinking and learning in nursing school. If you are an upper level nursing student or a student ready to graduate, this will serve as the basis for your job applications. This learning activity has two parts: Comparison, and Action Plan.

Comparison

Select two organizations you would consider as potential employers. Complete the Organization Comparison on Table 10.5.

Job search action plan

Develop a detailed timeline for your job search by completing Table 10.6 .

Table 10.5 Hospital comparison

Comparison element	Organization 1 _____	Organization 2 _____
Nurse residency program length, overview		
Magnet designation (yes/no)		
Quality ratings for Medicare (# of stars)		
Leapfrog quality ratings		
HCAHPS (Hospital Compare)		
Quality designations on hospital website		

Table 10.6 Job search action plan

Action	Date for completion
Write vision statement	
Create/update resume	
Compare potential employers	
Identify application requirements for employers I am interested in	
Identify potential references (list them)	
Attend nursing career fair	
Compile job application materials	
Contact references	
Schedule interviews	
Complete pre-employment screenings	

References

Banaszak-Holl, J., Castle, N. G., Lin, M. K., Shrivastwa, N., & Spreitzer, G. (2015). The role of organizational culture in retaining nursing workforce. *The Gerontologist, 55*(3), 462–471. https://doi.org/10.1093/geront/gnt129

Benner, P. (1982). From novice to expert. *American Journal of Nursing, 82*(3), 402–407.

Cunningham, T., Caza, B., Hayes, R., Leake, S., & Cipriano, P. (2024). Design health care systems to protect resilience in nursing. *Nursing Outlook, 72*(1), 101999. https://doi.org/10.1016/j.outlook.2023.101999

Goode, C. J., Glassman, K. S., Ponte, P. R., Krugman, M., & Peterson, T. (2018). Requiring a nurse residency for newly licensed registered nurses. *Nursing Outlook, 66*(3), 329–332. https://doi.org/10.1016/j.outlook.2018.04.004

Knighten, M. L. D. N.-B. (2022). New nurse residency programs: Benefits and return on investment. *Nursing Administration Quarterly, 46*(2), 185–190. https://doi.org/10.1097/NAQ.0000000000000522

Leep, L. K., & Stimpfel, A. W. (2024). A dimensional analysis of nursing unit culture. *Journal of Advanced Nursing, 80*(7), 2746–2757. https://doi.org/10.1111/jan.15985

U.S. Bureau of Labor Statistics. (2024, August 29). *Registered nurses: Occupational outlook handbook*. U.S. Bureau of Labor Statistics. Retrieved 20 Mar 2025 from https://www.bls.gov/ooh/healthcare/registered-nurses.htm

Webb, T., Parker, P., Huett, A., Weber, J., Harrison, T., & Nagel, C. (2024). The impact of nurse residency programs on patient quality and safety outcomes: A review of the literature. *Journal for Nurses in Professional Development, 40*(5), 268–272. https://doi.org/10.1097/NND.0000000000001058

NCLEX Essentials: From Application to Examination

11

The journey of a thousand miles begins with one step.

—*Lao Tzu*

11.1 Introduction

As you progress through nursing school, you'll hear the terms "NCLEX" and "NCLEX exam" mentioned frequently. The NCLEX exam is a milestone in your journey to becoming a licensed nurse. This chapter explains what you need to know about the NCLEX process, from application to examination. Understanding the NCLEX process early in your nursing education will help you approach your studies with purpose and prepare you for success on this critical exam.

▶ By the end of this chapter you will be able to:
1. Explain the purpose of the NCLEX and its role in nursing licensure.
2. Describe the NCLEX application process.
3. Identify the main content areas covered in the NCLEX exam.
4. Recognize different types of NCLEX questions, including Next Generation NCLEX (NGN) formats.
5. Understand the concept of Computer Adaptive Testing (CAT) and its impact on the NCLEX experience.

11.2 What Is NCLEX?

NCLEX® is an acronym for National Council Licensing Examination. It is called this because in the United States and Canada, every person who wants to become licensed as a Registered Nurse (RN) or Licensed Practical Nurse (LPN) has to complete an accredited nursing program,[1] then apply to licensure where they intend to have their first nursing job. The National Council of State Boards of Nursing (NCSBN) oversees the NCLEX exam.

11.2.1 The NCLEX Application Process

In each state and territory in the United States, or in each province and territory in Canada, a Nursing Regulatory Body (NRB) oversees licensure and practice. Your instructors will likely refer to the NRB as the "state board." For the purpose of clarity, in this chapter the term "state board" will be used to refer to the NRB.

---

[1] There are exceptions to this rule for completion of an accredited nursing program for applicants who have completed a nursing program in another country. Each State or Territory has rules about these application requirements.

© The Author(s), under exclusive license to Springer Nature Switzerland AG 2025
C. Thompson, *Nursing School, NCLEX and Career Transition Success*,
https://doi.org/10.1007/978-3-031-85538-2_11

When you decide where you will work after you graduate from your nursing program you will apply to that state board for licensure. You can apply for licensure in a state that is different from where you are in nursing school or your home state.

If you are in a nursing program in the United States, you may have heard about Nurse Compact Licensure (NCL), which allows nurses licensed in one NCL state to practice in another NCL state without going through the entire application process. Most States in the United States are NCL States. Don't be confused about what this means for you as a new nurse applying for licensure. You will need to apply for and obtain licensure in the state or territory where you plan to begin your first nursing position.

You can (and should) apply in your final semester or term of your nursing program. As you move through the application process, pay close attention to the details. You **must** follow the instructions and provide the exact documents required. Errors in your submission can result in processing delays you want to avoid.

While some students think it is better to wait until after graduation to apply for NCLEX, this is not recommended. You may experience delays in the processing of your application. You should plan to take NCLEX within 60 days of finishing your program, so you don't want to be held up by unexpected processing delays.

Let's look at the steps you will follow for your NCLEX.

- **Complete your licensure application**

The state board website will outline what you need to submit for your licensure application. Plan to

1. Create an account at the state board website.
2. Pay an application fee.
3. Submit identification documents.
4. Submit clearances such as FBI, Criminal Background, Child Abuse.
5. Submit Child Abuse training program completion certificate.

- **Your School of Nursing submits a verification of your education**

Your school of nursing will verify that you have completed the requirements for your nursing degree. Requirements for education verification submission vary and will be outlined on the state board website.

If you are applying for NCLEX as an international student or foreign nurse, you will need to refer to the state board website for instructions on documents required to verify your education and/or licensure.

- **Get your Authorization to Test (ATT)**

After you finish your nursing program, your application will be matched with the education verification that your school of nursing submitted. When those documents are matched and everything is in order, your state board will issue an Authorization to Test (ATT).

The ATT is an electronic approval that allows you to create an account with Pearson VUE. Upon receiving your ATT, you will get instructions for creating a Pearson VUE account. You will schedule your NCLEX exam at a Pearson Vue testing site through this account.

11.2.2 NCLEX Application: Plan in Advance

When you begin the application process, it is vital to have application documents in order so your ATT can be processed without delay. There are things that can hold up your application.

11.2.2.1 Mismatched Names

The name on your school transcript must be the same as your legal name. You will submit documentation of your legal name with your application. If you have changed your legal name, for example, if you got married during nursing school, be sure you change your name in your school system before your graduation. Otherwise, your application and your ATT will be delayed.

11.2.2.2 Previous Legal Charges

If you have criminal charges on your record, explore the impact of those charges on licensure. It is prudent to explore this well before your graduation.

11.2.2.3 Accommodation Requests

Each state board has requirements for accommodations requests. Specific instructions and forms for applying are in the state board website. Examples of accommodations include extended time, additional breaks, or separate testing room. You will need to submit a formal request and include documentation of your disability and a detailed explanation of the accommodations you are requesting.

Accommodation documentation is reviewed by the state board. Accommodation approval may change how you schedule your testing; however, instructions will be provided to you when the accommodations approval is sent.

11.2.2.4 Education Verification Discrepancies

If you are applying to a state board that is not familiar with your school of nursing, for example, you attended nursing school in Florida and decided to adventure to Alaska for your first nursing job, the Alaska State Board may require additional documentation from your Florida school to confirm you are completing your education requirements at an approved or legitimate nursing program.

Don't let this deter you from considering an adventure. Just plan and know that you may need to navigate the education verification process.

You can see the application process is complex and takes time. You don't want to put it off and risk delays in getting your ATT and scheduling your exam. Information and guidance on navigating this process are often incorporated into a course during your final semester.

11.2.2.5 The NCLEX Exam

Now that you understand what is involved for the NCLEX application in your final semester or term of nursing school, let's review what you need to know about your NCLEX exam. Your instructors in nursing school will often refer to NCLEX and because they understand it so well, may overlook explaining it.

The NCLEX exam is based on what a new nurse needs to know to practice safe and competent nursing care in entry level practice (NCSBN, 2023a). These competencies for entry level practice are outlined NCSBN for practical nurses (LPN/LVNs) (NCSBN, 2023b) and for registered nurses (RNs) (NCSBN, 2023a). For example, you may know when you finish nursing school you want to work as a nurse on a pediatric unit, however, you still need to demonstrate knowledge related to practice in any entry level setting.

Let's review this by looking at frequently asked questions about the exam.

How is entry level practice content identified?
NCSBN conducts job analysis to understand the tasks and responsibilities entry level nurses would be expected to perform in entry level practice settings (NCSBN, 2023a). As an example, operating room (OR) nursing is a specialized area of nursing practice that requires experience and additional training. OR nursing content is not on the NCLEX exam.

At regular intervals, NCSBN collects survey data from thousands of newly licensed nurses and from nurse administrators about entry level practice. Survey data is used to determine the NCLEX content, which is published in the NCLEX Test Plan (NCSBN, 2023a, b).

This Test Plan content is distributed by Client Needs Categories: (https://www.easynclex.com/review/the-distribution-of-questions-categories-on-nclex-rn-vs-nclex-pn-and-why.html).

Your nursing curriculum will not have been set up by Client Needs Categories, but the content will be woven into your courses, which are set up by topics (Fundamentals of Nursing, Pharmacology, Physical Assessment,

Pediatrics, Med/Surg, etc.) or by concepts or competencies (sample course names: Health and Wellness, Nursing Concepts 1, Nursing Concepts 2, Illness and Disease Management, Health Promotion and Disease Prevention). In either case, you can be assured your school of nursing has reviewed the Test Plan content and included it in your curriculum (the sequence of courses you take to graduate).

The focus of every question on the NCLEX exam is clinical judgment; you are given a scenario that an entry level nurse might encounter and select the response that reflects sound clinical judgment (what the nurse does) in the scenario. This is why critical thinking in your nursing school learning as outlined in Chap. 1 is pivotal to your NCLEX success.

Staying engaged in your learning using brain-based learning strategies and applying your growth mindset to your learning in every nursing course will help you to retain what you learn in your early nursing courses as you apply it in your upper level nursing courses and on NCLEX.

How is nursing school content covered in Client Needs Categories?

Nursing school content is distributed across the NCLEX Client Needs Categories ways that reflects the multifaceted nature of nursing care. This distribution ensures that nurses can apply their knowledge to various aspects of patient care, from safety and health promotion to complex physiological adaptations.

Let's use as an example the topic tuberculosis (TB) across Client Needs Categories.

1. Management of Care
   Coordinating a multidisciplinary discharge planning care team for a patient with Latent TB client.
2. Safety and Infection Control
   Implementing and maintaining airborne precautions for a client with active TB.
3. Health Promotion and Maintenance
   Educating family members of a TB client with Active TB about the importance of TB testing.

4. Psychosocial Integrity
   Addressing a client with Active TB expressions of anxiety and depression related to social isolation during the initial treatment.
5. Basic Care and Comfort
   Managing a client with Active TB persistent cough and fatigue, ensuring adequate rest, and maintaining proper nutrition to support recovery.
6. Pharmacological and Parenteral Therapies
   Monitoring the effectiveness and being aware of adverse effects of a multidrug regimen for TB treatment.
7. Reduction of Risk Potential
   Educating the patient about potential side effects and adverse effects of TB medications.
8. Physiological Adaptation
   Assessing and managing respiratory complications of Active TB.

These examples demonstrate how a single topic requires knowledge that spans all client needs categories. By organizing content this way, the NCLEX encourages you to think critically about client care from multiple angles. It's not just about knowing the facts of a topic but understanding how to apply that knowledge in different contexts and situations.

This approach aligns with principles of brain-based learning. By encountering the same topic in different contexts across your nursing education, you're engaging in spaced repetition and creating multiple neural pathways to access and apply this information. This not only helps with NCLEX preparation but also prepares you for the realities of nursing practice.

Adopting a growth mindset throughout your nursing education will help you see these interconnections and appreciate how each piece of knowledge contributes to your overall understanding of patient care. Rather than viewing each topic or category in isolation, integrate your learning across categories, just as you'll need to integrate different aspects of care for clients you encounter in your nursing practice.

What is covered in an "NCLEX review"?

You will likely be offered an NCLEX preparation course near the end of your program. The purpose of the preparation course is to outline the NCLEX testing format, Client Needs Categories, NCLEX question types, and test taking strategy.

The NCLEX review is not a comprehensive review of nursing school content. It teaches you how to apply the knowledge you already have. This is why embracing brain-based learning techniques throughout your program and applying a growth mindset to your learning is important for you to create your foundation of nursing knowledge.

Is NCLEX a multiple choice exam?

In each of your nursing classes you may have "NCLEX" questions for in-class review and on exams. In addition, you are likely to have an "NCLEX" product like Kaplan®, ATI®, or HESI® to supplement your NCLEX preparation. These will give questions in formats that are similar to NCLEX questions. Some of these are multiple choice questions but there are many other question types. You may hear these referred to as NGN questions.

Even though you will take "NCLEX" practice questions all through your nursing program, these questions are not typically as complex and difficult as questions you will see on the NCLEX exam.

NCLEX NGN Question Types

- Drag and drop
  - Order responses by what the nurse would do first, second, third, etc.
- Extended drag and drop
  - Order responses into more than one list of steps
- Drop down box
  - Selection of responses from a drop-down list
- Multiple choice
- Extended multiple response

- Like select all that apply but with more than five answer choices
- Highlight or Cloze
  - Select and highlight words or phrases that provide the nurse with priority information (cues) about the client
- Matrix grid
  - Select from a larger pool of options
- Bowtie items
  - Select and order answers into one of three categories: three in the first, two in the middle, and three in the third.
- Case Study

What is an NGN Case Study Question?

You will see *at least* three Case Study questions in your NCLEX exam. Each Case Study includes six questions that are based on the NCSBN's Clinical Judgement Measurement Model (Dickison et al., 2020). Created as a framework for measuring nurse's thinking, the Model overlaps with Tanner's Clinical Judgment Model, which you learned about in Chap. 1.

The six questions in each case study will follow the sequence of nurse's thinking and action based on this Measurement Model.

- **The first question tests your ability to recognize cues**:
  - Highlight assessment findings relevant to the presenting symptoms.
- **The second question tests your ability to analyze cues**.
  - Rank findings related to one diagnosis compared to another.
- **The third question tests your ability to prioritize hypotheses**.
  - Prioritize among findings
  - Identify risk potential for changes in the client's condition.
- **The fourth question tests how to generate solutions by taking a nursing action.**
  - Rank order nursing actions
  - Identify priority nursing action
- **The fifth question tests nursing actions**.
  - Identify steps to provide safe and effective care

- **The sixth question tests evaluation of outcomes.**
  - Discriminate between expected and unexpected client outcomes.

Understanding the sequence of NGN Case Study questions will help you to anticipate what to focus on as you move through the case study.

What is the Computer Adaptive Test (CAT)?
Another important thing to understand about NCLEX. It is a Computer Adaptive Test (CAT). This is a highly sophisticated testing format that is not scored based on overall percent.

Computer adaptive test means that the computer adjusts the questions you get based on how you answer each question. Each NCLEX question is ranked based on the degree of difficulty. The questions delivered on the exam are based on how you answer. When you answer a question correctly the next question you get will be a higher level of difficult question. On the other hand, when you miss a question you will "drop down" to a lower level question.

To pass NCLEX you need to demonstrate your ability to answer questions that are at or above the passing level for each Client Needs Category. With this format, you can't have weak areas and hope to avoid them on your NCLEX exam. The CAT format requires passing level mastery of content across every category. This is very important for you to understand because it means you will have to address your overall knowledge base and use test taking strategy so you don't miss questions due to reading errors or losing focus.

As you can see, the CAT testing format is complex and requires you to stay on top of your learning throughout nursing school, not plan to "brush up" on everything at the end.

This highlights key aspects of the NCLEX exam that every nursing student should understand. From the breakdown of content categories to the types of questions you'll encounter, and the unique computer adaptive testing format, each element plays a crucial role in your NCLEX experience. NCLEX is designed to test your ability to apply nursing knowledge across various scenarios, not just recall facts. Approaching your exam preparation with the critical thinking, brain-based learning, and growth mindset strategies you've learned in this book will prepare you to be successful when you take NCLEX.

11.3 Conclusion

Building your NCLEX knowledge base throughout your nursing program is the key to a painless NCLEX success journey. A fixed mindset in nursing school, with a focus on merely passing each assignment or course, is a detriment to NCLEX success. Applying critical thinking to your learning, integrating brain-based learning, adopting a growth mindset, and embracing the strategies outlined in this book will not only prepare you for the NCLEX but also launch you toward a successful and fulfilling nursing career. Your dedication and hard work will pave the way for you to achieve your dreams and make a significant impact in the field of nursing.

If you are in your final semester or term of your nursing program, the next two chapters will be essential reading for you to be prepared for NCLEX success. You will learn what you need to focus on in your final semester. Keeping in mind that your final NCLEX preparation will occur after you graduate, the final chapter in Part III outlines the work you will need to do to take you from graduation to NCLEX success.

Chapter 11 Synthesis Learning Activity: NCLEX Application Plan
The purpose of this assignment is to help you understand and prepare for the NCLEX application process, regardless of where you are in your nursing education journey.

Visit the website for the Nurse Regulatory Body (State Board) where you plan to apply for licensure. Complete Table 11.1 Application Information and Timeline.

Know what to expect for your budget. If you are completing this well in advance of your graduation from nursing school, anticipate that some of the costs may increase. Complete Table 11.2 Costs for Licensure.

Table 11.1 Nurse Regulatory Board (State Board) application information

Category	Requirements	Planned date for completion
Creating an account		
Required application documents (list them)		
Criminal background check		
Child abuse education		
Requirements for accommodations (if applicable)		
Education verification		

Table 11.2 Costs for licensure

Category	Cost	Payment method
Application fee		
Background checks		
Fingerprinting (if applicable)		
NCLEX registration fee		
Other required documents (list)		

References

Dickison, P., Haerling, K. A., & Lasater, K. (2020). NCSBN clinical judgment measurement model clarification. *Journal of Nursing Education, 59*(7), 365–365. https://doi.org/10.3928/01484834-20200617-02

NCSBN. (2023a). *Next generation NCLEX® NCLEX-RN® effective April 2023*. Retrieved November 5, 2024 from https://www.nclex.com/files/2023_RN_Test%20Plan_English_FINAL.pdf

NCSBN. (2023b). *Next generation NCLEX® NCLEX-PN® effective April 2023*. Retrieved November 5, 2024 from https://www.nclex.com/files/2023_PN_Test%20Plan_FINAL.pdf

Preparing for NCLEX in Your Final Semester

12

It always seems impossible until it's done.

—*Nelson Mandela*

12.1 Introduction

Your final semester (or term) of nursing school is an exciting time, filled with anticipation of graduation and starting your nursing career. However, it's also a critical period for NCLEX preparation. This chapter will guide you through your final semester and provide strategies to maximize your preparation while maintaining a growth mindset.

▶ **By the end of this chapter you will be able to:**
1. Understand the purpose and components of final semester NCLEX preparation.
2. Distinguish between common myths and realities of NCLEX prep.
3. Apply strategies to maintain a growth mindset throughout your final semester.
4. Navigate professional communication for conflict resolution.

12.2 Your Final Semester

If you are reviewing this chapter early in your nursing career you may want to revisit and read it again when you are beginning your final semester.

If you are in your final semester, congratulations! You are on the home stretch. After all of your hard work, you are near the end.

You have much to look forward to: finishing nursing school, starting your nursing career, having an income that exceeds your expenses, and planning for this next big phase of your life. Staying focused on the present, especially NCLEX prep, can be challenging amid the excitement. However, dedicating time and effort to your NCLEX preparation is crucial.

Completing your NCLEX assignments with a growth mindset will contribute to your success. This means that you will embrace the learning in each of your assigned activities. This can be challenging as it will be a busy semester!

If you have used critical thinking, brain-based learning, and a growth mindset throughout your nursing program, the NCLEX practice questions you review in this final semester will "wake up" stored memories. You will now apply that knowledge.

© The Author(s), under exclusive license to Springer Nature Switzerland AG 2025
C. Thompson, *Nursing School, NCLEX and Career Transition Success*,
https://doi.org/10.1007/978-3-031-85538-2_12

Table 12.1 NCLEX myth vs reality

Myth	Reality
The NCLEX live review course at the end of the final semester will review the content I need to know for NCLEX	The NCLEX live review teaches you how to APPLY what you have learned to NCLEX type questions, you will not review all of your nursing school content
I have taken NCLEX questions all through nursing school so I won't need days of review to learn that	Questions on exams have been difficult and many were even NGN style questions. However, they were not NCLEX questions. NCLEX questions are higher level questions that are more difficult than what you typically see in your nursing exams
I will be ready to take NCLEX when I graduate	Some students may be able to take NCLEX right after graduation but this is not the norm. Most nursing school graduates will need to spend NCLEX prep time after graduation in order to be successful on NCLEX
If you pass the end of program NCLEX readiness test you will pass NCLEX	You will have a benchmark score on NCLEX readiness tests. If you meet the benchmark you will need to continue question practice as you wait for your NCLEX test date. If you score below the benchmark, you will need to be diligent about using your NCLEX practice tests to identify and fill in your knowledge gaps. Either way, you will need to plan to do additional work to prepare for NCLEX after you graduate

12.2.1 NCLEX: Testing Your Ability to Think Like a Nurse

Preparing for NCLEX is not separate from preparing for nursing practice. The exam is designed to test your ability to think critically with each question. Each question tests your ability to make the correct choice about nursing action (clinical judgments) that represent how nurses think and apply clinical decision making to practice.

As you engage with NCLEX prep material integrate your learning into your practice of thinking like a nurse. Use critical thinking when analyzing questions and selecting answers. Apply clinical decision making and judgment to each scenario and view each question as an opportunity to reinforce your nursing knowledge and skills.

Practice critical thinking and keep a positive attitude to support your learning.

12.2.2 Final Semester NCLEX Preparation: MYTHS Versus REALITY

Table 12.1 outlines myths and misunderstandings that you are likely to hear in nursing school.

Pause and Reflect 12.1: My NCLEX Journey

Take a few moments to reflect on your current understanding and feelings about NCLEX preparation. Whether you're early in your nursing education or approaching graduation, this reflection will help you identify beliefs and attitudes that may impact your NCLEX preparation journey.

1. What I've Heard About NCLEX
   List two to three things you've heard about NCLEX. This could be things you've heard from other nursing students, nursing instructors, nurses you've met, social media, or from other sources.
2. NCLEX Reality Check.
   Review Table 12.1 NCLEX Myths and Realities. For each item you listed in #1, answer the following:
   Is it a myth or reality based on what you've learned?
   What evidence or information supports or refutes what you heard?
   How does this new understanding impact your approach to NCLEX preparation?

(continued)

3. My NCLEX Mindset

Write your reflection for each of the following prompts:

Right now, my biggest concern about NCLEX is...

One thing I can do now to support my future NCLEX success is...

When I hear others talking about NCLEX, I will...

4. Commitment to Growth Mindset for NCLEX Success

Write a brief statement about how you will maintain a growth mindset in your NCLEX preparation journey. If you're early in your program, focus on how you'll approach learning with NCLEX in mind. If you're in your final semester, focus on specific actions you'll take to prepare.

12.3 What to Expect in Your Final Semester NCLEX Preparation

Most nursing programs integrate NCLEX preparation activities and assignments, including a live review course, into the final semester or term in nursing school. These might be included in a course as graded or ungraded assignments, or be assigned in addition to required coursework.

You will also most likely be using an NCLEX preparation product. In many cases you have used this product throughout the program, and in this final semester will be using the resources in the product that are specific to end of program NCLEX preparation.

You are likely to see the following assignments:

- **NCLEX assessment test in the beginning of the semester**

This test will show where you stand in terms of your NCLEX knowledge base as you begin your final NCLEX prep.

This test consists of high level application questions on all nursing program content. If you applied brain-based learning and critical thinking throughout your learning, you will be able to recall much of the information for this test.

This test has a "benchmark" score. If you are above the benchmark, that means your knowledge base **coming into the final semester** is where it should be. This doesn't mean you are ready for NCLEX, it just means you are on track to continue your NCLEX prep.

If you are below the benchmark, that means your knowledge base is not where it should be. Sadly, your final semester is going to be too busy to fill in major knowledge gaps from your previous courses. However, you can make the most of it by really applying yourself to learning content as you complete your NCLEX prep assignments throughout the semester.

- **Weekly NCLEX question sets**

You may be required to take a certain amount of questions from the question bank each week and remediate those tests. This is how you will build your knowledge base throughout the semester and will decrease the burden of postgraduation NCLEX prep.

The primary goal of your weekly practice is to enhance the interleaving of content as you prepare for NCLEX. The repetition and "chunking" of your learning is contributing to your success. Approach it with a growth mindset, not a fixed mindset.

- **NCLEX Live Review course**

An NCLEX Live Review will likely be scheduled near the end of your final semester and offered with one of your nursing instructors, an outside instructor, or as a virtual course.

The Live Review is not a content review. If you did not bring a good foundation of content knowledge into your final semester, you will need to bring your knowledge base up to speed during the semester and as you continue your preparation after graduation.

For many students, the Live Review course falls during a time when you are overwhelmed with multiple priorities; finishing required coursework, planning for graduation and a possible move, as well as your job search. The Live Review can feel like something to sit through (fixed mindset—get it over with) rather than a learning experience (growth mindset). A fixed mindset during your Live Review is an NCLEX success landmine. Be mindful and focused throughout the Live Review. It is a foundation for your success.

- **NCLEX readiness test**

Different from the NCLEX assessment test you took at the beginning of the semester, the readiness test consists of higher level NCLEX type questions like you have seen in the weekly question sets. You should be assigned to take this test after the live review so that you can apply the strategies you learned in the live review.

The benchmark on this test correlates with readiness to pass NCLEX. If you meet the benchmark, this means following your NCLEX prep product recommended practice test sequences after graduation should prepare you for NCLEX. If you continue to meet the benchmarks, you will be ready.

If you score below the benchmark, you will need to be diligent about your postgraduation. Refer to Chap. 13 for detailed guidance on this.

Nursing School Application: Time Management: Three Paths Through Final Semester NCLEX

Lucia's Story: Catching Up From Behind

Throughout nursing school, Lucia juggled many outside responsibilities. While she managed to pass her courses, her learning often focused on immediate course requirements rather than building a strong knowledge foundation. Entering her final semester, her initial NCLEX assessment score was low, and she needed to focus her attention on passing her courses. Rather than becoming discouraged, she made a realistic assessment of her situation. She recognized that her approach to nursing school—doing just enough to pass each course—had left her with significant knowledge gaps to address. She decided not to apply for nursing positions immediately after graduation, instead planning dedicated time for intensive NCLEX preparation.

Ravi's Story: Steady Progress

Ravi learned after a few first semester missteps the importance of applying a growth mindset and improving his student behaviors to support his success. When he repeated his first nursing clinical course, he focused on applying critical thinking, brain-based learning strategies, and a growth mindset and saw how that contributed to his success. He wasn't a top performer but he was comfortable able to pass his courses and progress through the nursing major. In his final semester, despite his roommates' frequent invitations to relax and enjoy "senior slide," Ravi stayed committed to his NCLEX preparation assignments. With his dream job offer contingent on passing NCLEX within 6 weeks of graduation, he knew every practice question and review session mattered. His end-of-program assessment scored just above the benchmark—exactly where he hoped to be. He was on track to meet his goals; passing NCLEX within 6 weeks of graduation.

Ana's Story: Managing High Expectations

Ana's strong academic performance throughout nursing school reflected her dedicated approach to learning. Not naturally gifted at test-taking, she compensated

(continued)

12.3 What to Expect in Your Final Semester NCLEX Preparation

with attention to applying her critical thinking and growth mindset as she progressed through her nursing program. Her initial NCLEX assessment scores were well above benchmark and she was on track to graduate with a firm footing in her knowledge base and prepared to pass NCLEX with minimal postgraduation work.

Each of these student's story highlights the importance of realistic self-assessment and appropriate action based on individual circumstances.

12.3.1 Maintaining a Growth Mindset Throughout Your Final Semester

As you can see, you are likely to have a variety of NCLEX prep assignments in addition to other coursework you will be completing during your final semester. It is important for you to maintain your growth mindset, embracing this work that is essential for your success.

When you use a growth mindset you reframe challenges as opportunities. Instead of viewing the NCLEX prep assignments as a burden, see it as a chance to reinforce your knowledge and improve your critical thinking skills. Each practice question becomes an opportunity to learn and grow.

Embrace the process of learning. When you begin with NCLEX practice questions you may not score well. Don't get discouraged but see this as a ladder of growth.

Consciously staying connected with your growth mindset practice will support your learning along the way and contribute to your NCLEX success.

Pause and Reflect 12.2: Seeing My Path to NCLEX Success

1. Review Naomi, Ravi, and Alba's stories from Nursing School Application: Three Paths Through Final Semester NCLEX Preparation. Consider your study habits throughout nursing school, current knowledge base, outside responsibilities, and postgraduation plans.

   Which student's approach most closely matches your current path? Why?

2. Complete Table 12.2 to reflect on your Preparation Self-Assessment.

3. Planning My Path Forward. Based on your reflections in Table 12.2 Preparation Self-Assessment consider the following.

   What adjustments (if any) do you need to make to your current approach?

   Time management

   Study strategies

   Using critical thinking

   Commitment to growth mindset learning

Table 12.2 Preparation self-assessment

Preparation area	Strong	Developing	Needs improvement
Understanding of foundational nursing concepts			
Consistency in study habits			
Balance of school and other responsibilities			
Test-taking strategies			
Critical thinking skills			
Ability to commit to growth mindset for learning			

12.3.2 Be Professional If the Work Is Too Much

If you are finding it difficult to attend to your growth mindset because of overwhelming course demands, consider speaking with course faculty. This is an opportunity to develop professional conflict resolution skills. Here are some tips for you to consider:

- **Address your concern without joining in other students' complaints.**

This is a challenge you may encounter in your role as a professional nurse. For example, your nurse manager may add workload responsiblity that is not feasible or safe. Rather than complain with your co-workers, a professional approach is to navigate resolution using positive communication. In professional practice, and as a nursing student, is it prudent to avoid joining in on complaint sessions.

- **Follow the "chain of command."**

Chain of command means you address a concern with the person directly responsible rather than going above that person in the organizational structure. Speak first to the instructors, not to a program administrator such as the Dean or the Chairperson.

Begin your discussion about the issue with the course faculty who assigned the work. If you do not get resolution then you go higher. If the work is spread over more than one course, speak with each course faculty without pitting one against the other.

- **Be professional in your request to meet.**

If possible, approach the instructor in person during office hours or request a meeting by email. Don't approach the instructor before or after class with an important issue like this. You are showing respect by not blindsiding the instructor with the topic in a public setting in front of other students.

Be professional in this initial request for a meeting and have your talking points ready. If you send the request by email, begin with the proper salutation; Dr. Jones, Professor Jones, Instructor Jones.

If you are composing an email to request a meeting, make it professional. You can even use AI to edit and check your professionalism. Don't begin the email with "Hey" or with the instructor's first name. Close your email with a sign-off like "Respectfully" before your name.

- **Be responsible for this concern as your concern.**

Your instructor will bristle when you begin with "all of the students" or "other students asked me to talk to you." Ganging up on your instructor sets up an aggressive tone. Take responsibility. You can add "I may speak for other students as well, but I know that for me....."

- **Be prepared for your meeting with positive, nonaggressive talking points.**

Remember your basics of positive communication. Avoid "you" statements like "you have assigned too much work." and frame your comments using "I" statements.

Begin with an introduction such as: "I understand this work is very important for NCLEX and for my nursing practice. I want to do my best."

Continue with your main points "I find when I am looking at the due dates and trying to get it all done I am not able to attend to it all without compromising on my learning."

End with a succinct summary of your request. "I am hoping you'd consider a way to look over the work we have due for the remainder of the semester and see if there are any assignments that could be altered to reduce the overall workload."

- **Show respect for your instructor's expertise.**

Typically, when you are approaching conflict resolution in a professional way, you want to include potential solutions. However, in this case, your instructor is the expert on course content and learning competencies to be met in final semester courses. You do not want to make suggestions about assignments to be eliminated because you don't have the level of knowledge and expertise to weigh in on these choices.

Following these guidelines will help you practice professional conflict resolution skills. Hopefully if you find yourself in a situation of having to use this strategy, this approach will yield a good outcome for you.

Nursing School Application: Professional Communication in Action: Ana's Approach

Ana was committed to her final semester NCLEX preparation work, but when one of her final semester course instructors began adding weekly assignments that overlapped with scheduled NCLEX preparation deadlines, Ana was stressed about keeping up. Students were complaining among themselves about these additional assignments. Rather than joining these complaints, Ana decided to address the situation professionally. She composed a carefully worded email to her instructor:

Subject: Request for Meeting Regarding Course Workload.

Dear Professor Copeland,

I am writing to request a brief meeting with you to discuss the course assignments and NCLEX preparation requirements. I am committed to doing my best work in both areas and would appreciate your guidance in managing these concurrent responsibilities.

Would you have availability during your office hours this week to meet?

Thank you for considering my request.

Respectfully,
Ana Pasthel.

During the meeting, Ana maintained a professional approach. She began by acknowledging the value of both the course content and NCLEX preparation: "I understand these assignments help prepare us for nursing practice, and I want to learn as much as I can. I'm finding it challenging to give both the coursework and NCLEX preparation the attention they deserve."

Rather than suggesting specific solutions, Ana shared her concern about compromising learning in either area: "I want to be sure I'm getting the most out of both experiences. I'm wondering if you could help me think through how to manage these competing demands."

Professor Copeland appreciated Ana's professional approach and concern for learning. After their discussion, she reviewed the assignment schedule and recognized the overlap in due dates. At the next class meeting, she announced a revised schedule alternating weekly between course assignments and NCLEX preparation work.

Ana's approach demonstrated the effectiveness of addressing concerns constructively rather than joining in complaints. She focused on learning outcomes rather than workload complaints, respected her instructor's expertise, and this brought about a solution that benefited everyone.

You may not have any difficulty managing your NCLEX assignments during your last semester, but you are likely to have had a conflict at some point during nursing school. Conflict resolution is a valuable skill for professionals. Complete the Pause and Reflect 12.3 to review this topic.

Table 12.3 Professional conflict resolution

Element of professional communication	Present in my approach? Yes/No	How could I improve?
Avoided "joining in" group complaining		
Followed appropriate "chain of command"		
Maintained professional behavior in verbal and non-verbal communication		
Prepared before communication		
Took responsibility for the concern		
Remained assertive, not aggressive		
Respected authority and expertise of person in charge		

Pause and Reflect 12.3: Developing Professional Conflict Resolution Skills

Think about a time you needed to resolve a conflict in an academic or professional setting. Compare your approach to Ana's professional communication strategies by completing Table 12.3 Professional Conflict Resolution.

What would you do differently if faced with a similar situation now?

Professional communication skills, like NCLEX preparation, develop through conscious practice and a growth mindset. The case studies show how the final semester presents various challenges with NCLEX preparation while you are completing your final semester coursework. Whether you find yourself needing to focus primarily on building your knowledge, maintaining steady, or working to continue to excel, your success depends on embracing the work. You won't complete your final semester fully prepared for NCLEX. Additional preparation after graduation is a given, but how much work you'll need to do depends on how well you use your final semester preparation time.

12.4 Conclusion

Your final semester is a crucial time for NCLEX preparation. By understanding the purpose of the process and assignments, maintaining a growth mindset, and using your critical thinking to assess your needs at this time will help you make the most of this preparation period. The goal is not just to pass NCLEX, but to develop the critical thinking and clinical judgment skills that will serve you throughout your nursing career. Stay focused, embrace the challenge, and trust in the preparation you've done throughout your nursing education.

In the next chapter, you will review the NCLEX preparation to plan for after your graduation or program completion.

Preparing for NCLEX After Graduation

13

By failing to prepare, you are preparing to fail.

—*Benjamin Franklin*

13.1 Introduction

Whether you're approaching graduation or have recently completed nursing school, NCLEX preparation is an ongoing process. This chapter provides a comprehensive, step-by-step approach to NCLEX preparation along with tools to help you gauge your readiness. By following these guidelines, you'll develop the knowledge base and critical thinking skills needed to pass NCLEX, as you build the confidence you need to manage anxiety when you take NCLEX. Through systematic preparation, you'll know exactly when you're ready to test. While you may find reviewing this chapter helpful during nursing school to understand post-graduation needs, you'll want to revisit it when actively preparing for NCLEX to guide your preparation journey.

▶ **By the end of this chapter you will be able to:**
1. Develop a realistic timeline for NCLEX preparation after graduation.
2. Select and utilize appropriate NCLEX prep resources.
3. Implement effective study strategies for knowledge retention.

4. Use critical thinking to analyze and improve your test-taking performance.
5. Overcome NCLEX test anxiety.

13.2 Understanding the NCLEX Preparation Journey

If you are still in your nursing program, you will be hearing about NCLEX preparation with each course. The focus during nursing school is on building on your knowledge base as you learn to apply critical thinking to nursing practice decisions. This builds the foundation for your NCLEX preparedness.

In the last semester or term of your program, you will most likely have a systematic approach with activities and assignments for NCLEX preparation integrated into a course. The framework of what this most likely consists of is reviewed in Chap. 12. Some students perform well enough in their final semester work that they need only minimal additional preparation between graduation and taking the NCLEX.

However, many students—in fact, most—will need more than just minimal practice before test day. This chapter will guide you through effective

© The Author(s), under exclusive license to Springer Nature Switzerland AG 2025
C. Thompson, *Nursing School, NCLEX and Career Transition Success*,
https://doi.org/10.1007/978-3-031-85538-2_13

145

13.2.1 The Reality of Postgraduation NCLEX Preparation

Many students and their families ask, "After all this time in nursing school, aren't you ready to take the NCLEX?" It's a valid question, but the reality is more complex.

Nursing school provides you with the foundation needed for safe and effective entry-level nursing practice. However, like many other professions requiring licensure, additional preparation is necessary to succeed on the licensing exam.

Many nursing school graduates do not understand the level of postgraduation preparation needed for NCLEX success. Even though around 90% of first time test takers will pass (NCSBN, 2025), you want to do everything you can to prevent falling into the 10% who do not pass on their first attempt.

13.2.2 Why Passing NCLEX on Your First Attempt Matters

You can retake the NCLEX if you are not successful on your first attempt. Depending on the Nursing Regulatory Board (or State Board of Nursing as it is commonly known) where you are applying for licensure, you may have a limited number of attempts before you have to take a review program. Most State Boards will allow you an unlimited number of attempts with a 45 day wait period between attempts.

However, there are several compelling reasons why you should strive to pass on your first attempt. Most nursing school graduates who do not pass on their first attempt have difficulty passing on their next attempt. Retest pass rates are less than 50% (NCSBN, 2025). Studies have documented the negative impact of NCLEX failure on mental health and well-

being that impacts retest success (Claudette, 2014; Kasprovich & VandeVusse, 2018; Poorman & Webb, 2000). This emotional setback creates challenges for maintaining the confidence necessary to be successful in future attempts.

In addition to the emotional setback, not passing NCLEX on your first attempt may impact the nursing position you have accepted. The job offer could be rescinded, or if you have been hired as a GN (graduate nurse) a demotion until you pass on retest.

In every state board jurisdiction, NCLEX failure results in a 45-day wait before retesting. This means that if you don't pass, you can't go the following week to retest. This delay exacerbates the financial impact of not passing.

Preparing to pass on your first attempt is what you want to strive for. There is no shortcut to NCLEX prep.

13.2.3 When Should I Plan to Take NCLEX?

You should take the NCLEX as soon as you are ready, but not *before* you are ready. It is best to take it within 60 days of graduation.

Depending on where you are applying for licensure you may be able to begin work as a Graduate Nurse (GN) but be cautious about overcommitting yourself to work hours. It is tempting to finally have this opportunity for income, however, don't let that get in the way of making time for your prep.

Nursing School Application: Postgraduation NCLEX Preparation
Nursing School Application: Two NCLEX Prep Approaches

Case Study 1: Jordan's Overconfidence

Jordan did well in nursing school. He typically did well on his exams even though

(continued)

he worked two 8-h shifts per week while he was in nursing school. Critical thinking came easily to him; he was often able to do well without rigorous study time.

His end-of-program NCLEX readiness assessment results were strong, boosting his confidence further. After graduation, Jordan took a 4-week break from studying, believing he was well-prepared for the NCLEX.

When Jordan resumed his NCLEX prep, he found his motivation and momentum had waned. He would open his NCLEX prep account, attempt a few practice questions, but then get distracted and stop studying. Jordan downloaded an NCLEX question app and when he was bored, he'd take a few questions and review the rationale. He didn't track a cumulative score in this app but he felt he was doing well and he had already scheduled his NCLEX exam.

On test day, Jordan rushed through the questions, still confident in his abilities. As the exam continued past 100 questions he began to lose confidence. By the time he reached 145 questions, Jordan had lost all focus. He had not "trained" his brain for this long test. He may have had some knowledge gaps but his inability to stay focused for this long a test was most likely the biggest factor that led to his NCLEX failure.

Case Study 2: Sonya's Structured Approach

Sonya's end-of-program NCLEX readiness test results were below the passing benchmark. This didn't surprise her. During nursing school Sonya achieved passing grades without excelling because her work schedule during nursing school forced her to shift from a growth to a fixed mindset in many of her courses. She had to prioritize assignment completion over learning. After graduation, Sonya continued working two 12-h shifts per week as a CNA in the med-surg unit where she had accepted an RN position pending NCLEX success.

Sonya created a structured NCLEX prep plan that included:

- A prep calendar with scheduled study time on her days off.
- Reducing her social media activity.
- Letting family and friends know about her "phone-free" study periods.
- Continued practice in the NCLEX prep product, following the recommended sequence of practice tests.
- Applied active learning and critical thinking strategies to understand content and apply it to thinking like a nurse when she approached practice questions.
- Monitored her progress, noting steady improvement in her scores.

After scoring above the benchmark on four consecutive exams, she scheduled her NCLEX, giving herself 4 weeks for continued preparation. She used this time to create practice tests in her weakest client needs categories, reviewing missed questions using active learning techniques to be sure she learned and understood the content.

In the days leading up to her exam, she felt relaxed and confident, knowing she had prepared thoroughly and strategically. She passed NCLEX on her first attempt.

These case studies illustrate the importance of structured, consistent preparation and the potential pitfalls of overconfidence in NCLEX preparation. They also demonstrate how applying critical thinking, brain-based learning, and a growth mindset can lead to more effective NCLEX preparation, even when balancing work and study commitments.

13.2.4 Be Realistic About How Much Time You Need for NCLEX Prep

End of program assessments are very reliable, however, because it is given at the end of your nursing program when you had other priorities, you may have not been able to do your best.

How did you score on the end of program assessment compared to the passing or "ready" benchmark?

At, just below, or just above benchmark. If your score was at, just below, or just above the benchmark (for example, benchmark was 63% and your score was somewhere between 60 and 64%) consider factors that may have affected your score:

- Did you take the assessment test:
    - After completing a different course exam?
    - After working a night shift or a night of poor sleep?
    - Without doing your best or caring about your performance?
    - When your mind was other places?

If you answered yes to any of the questions, it is likely you could have scored well above the benchmark. However, you don't have a way to predict how much not being at your best impacted your overall score. Be cautious about using "I know I would have done better if…" as a reason to short cut your postgraduate prep.

Well below benchmark. While the factors above may have impacted your score, coming in below benchmark suggests you will need to commit to NCLEX prep time to address knowledge and test-taking strategies. You may make quick progress, or you may have knowledge gaps that will take time to address.

Well above benchmark. Good for you! This will give you confidence for your NCLEX prep and sticking to your prep. Using QBanks to guide your progress, you should be confident in your ability to test within 60 days of graduation.

Now that you understand more about the postgraduation NCLEX preparation journey, complete Pause and Reflect 13.1 to analyze your needs.

Pause and Reflect 13.1: Analyzing your NCLEX Preparation Approach

1. Review your end of program NCLEX readiness assessment score. Was it below, at, or above benchmark. What does your score tell you about your needs for postgraduation NCLEX preparation work?
2. You read in the Nursing School Application—Postgraduation NCLEX Preparation about Jordan and Sonya's approaches to postgraduation NCLEX preparation. Evaluate your preparation needs by completing Table 13.1.

Understanding your preparation needs and plan will help you as you move forward with

Table 13.1 Preparation self-assessment

Preparation element	(Yes/no)	How to improve
I have created a structured study schedule based on my readiness test performance		
I have a realistic plan to balance work and other commitments with NCLEX preparation time		
I approach each practice test as a learning opportunity, taking time to understand content rather than just reviewing answers		
I commit to focused practice sessions without distractions		
I apply a growth mindset to my test review. I take time to learn and understand content instead of passively reading answer rationale		
I commit to taking each practice test with focus to do my best		
I have a plan for preparation that will reduce my NCLEX test anxiety		
I am building confidence through systematic preparation rather than relying on past performance		

13.3 📝 Practical Strategies: Postgraduation NCLEX Preparation

your postgraduation work. Let's look at some practical strategies that will help you as you move forward with an NCLEX preparation product that will support your work.

Table 13.2 NCLEX product do's and don'ts

Do	Don't
Use a reliable product. There are many on the market and they are priced competitively	Share a product with another person. You need to track your own progress
Select a product that lets you track progress by Client Needs Category	Use free testing resources; they are not likely to have valid NCLEX practice questions
Trust the resource. You will get an overall prediction of your readiness that is reliable	Use multiple products. You can track your progress using one product

- **Select an NCLEX prep product**

  The product you used in school; it may have been Kaplan®, ATI®, HESI®, NurseThink®, or another product, will have NCLEX Qbanks for you to create practice tests. It will also have NCLEX readiness assessment and CAT tests.

  You don't need to purchase another product. This product you had in school will have a sufficient number of questions to practice and monitor your progress. In addition, this product will have other resources such as videos and test rationales to help you fill in your knowledge gaps.

  Some students, by the time they finish nursing school are DONE with the product they used in school. They may have had frustrating experiences not meeting the benchmark on tests, or maybe had burdensome test remediation requirements in nursing school. In addition, learning styles are unique. Some students just don't connect with the format or layout of the product and get frustrated using it.

  Remember that attitude influences learning. If you can't shake your bad attitude about the product you may consider purchasing something else. However, if finances are limited and the product itself works for you, you just don't like it, try adjusting your attitude. Try saying "I'm on the home stretch and I can say goodbye to this!"

  If you decide to purchase or use a different product review Table 13.2 Product Do's and Don'ts for tips on what to select.

- **Familiarize yourself with the NCLEX prep platform and resources**

When you completed your NCLEX live review, you should have been given information about each of the features for the product you used in school. If you are using that or if you purchased something else be sure you know:

- The product benchmark for determining NCLEX readiness.
- Where to find content review resources.
- How to build question banks.
- How to track your overall progress.
- Where to find your overall scores for each Client Needs Category.

NCLEX prep products will also include different types of **QBanks**.

- Readiness Tests (may be called Assessment Tests).
  - Include NCLEX Client Needs Categories in the proportion seen in NCLEX.
  - Includes NGN questions in the proportion seen in NCLEX.
- Computer Adaptive Tests (CAT) tests
  - Deliver questions based on performance. (See to CAT testing review in this chapter).
  - Number of questions varies depending on performance.
  - Final score shows a readiness prediction.
  - Includes NGN questions in the proportion seen in NCLEX.
- NCLEX QBanks.
  - Tests you build.

- You create by selecting:
  Number of questions.
  Areas of content.
  Client Needs Category.
  Unused questions.
  NGN or standard NCLEX questions.
- NGN QBanks
  - Composed only of NGN questions.

- **Follow the product's NCLEX success plan**

The product will lay out a plan for you to follow. Just like you should trust the product, trust the product plan. Even if you scored well in your final semester practice tests, continue practice and follow the recommended sequence for practice tests. Once you pass NCLEX, you won't even have to do practice tests again. Keep that in mind if you're feeling test fatigue.

- **Focus on improving your focus**

There is no shortcut to teaching your brain to stay focused. The strategies outlined in Chap. 4 include information about the value of mind relaxation for improving your focus. Hopefully you were able to apply that throughout nursing school. If not, now is the time to get serious about cutting down on distractions (yes, that means your cell phone and social media.)

- **Take every practice test in test mode, not tutor mode**

You will learn best if you use test mode. Complete each test and then go back and review your results. Taking tests one question at a time and reviewing the rationale after each question is a passive learning strategy that is not likely to improve your knowledge retention. In addition, this strategy does not prepare your brain for the actual NCLEX test.

- **Use each practice test to identify content you need to learn**

After you have completed each test, take a break, then go back and review each question.

Use active learning strategies to teach yourself the question content you did not know. Even if you answered correctly but guessed, review that content in a way that you learn AND understand.

- **Handwrite content review notes for every question topic you did not know**

You will make progress and see your scores improve when you learn content then apply that learning to future questions on the content.

Handwriting processes your learning more effectively than simply reading the rationale (this is passive learning) and more effectively than typing or cutting and pasting the notes in your computer.

- **Take every practice test as if it were your NCLEX**

Set aside at least 3 h for practice test sessions. Go to a quiet place where you can take the test without interruptions. Yes, this means leaving your phone and smartwatch behind.

If you take a prepared practice test (one included in the product as an assessment test) or a CAT test you will be taking at least 85 questions. If you create your own practice test using QBank questions, create an 85 question test.

This is important because you are using your practice test scores to prepare for your exam and to predict your readiness. If you don't score well on a practice test because you were distracted, you can't know how much the distraction impacted your performance.

- **Include practice tests that have more than 85 questions**

Your goal of course is to do your best on the NCLEX, which is reflected by having the exam stop at 85 questions with a pass. However, even the most prepared students experience test day nerves. While you want to hope you'll have just 85 questions, you need to plan for the possibility of the exam going up to the maximum of 150 questions.

13.3 Practical Strategies: Postgraduation NCLEX Preparation

The CAT testing format requires focus for the duration of the exam. If you have gone beyond 85 questions, each time you miss a passing level question you drop below the passing benchmark for the entire exam. You need to be above passing level in every Client Needs Category. Being just below passing level in one Client Needs Category will result in your not passing the exam.

Many students who take NCLEX and don't pass at 150 questions will admit that by the end, they were stressed out, discouraged, and no longer able to stay focused. This is a circumstance you can prevent by "training" yourself to stay focused in longer practice exam sessions.

- **Keep a positive attitude and mindset**

Stay focused on your self-talk; it is just as important now as it was in nursing school. Review the self-talk in Tables 13.2 and 13.3.

- **Monitor practice test scores**

As you follow this process of taking tests, reviewing the content, writing remediation study notes, reviewing those notes (brain-based learning), and taking more practice tests, you should see your test scores improve. If they are not improving, review the next section in this chapter on Test Analysis to identify how to improve.

- **Plan to take NCLEX when you are CONSISTENTLY scoring above the product's readiness benchmark in every test and in every Client Needs Category.**

There will be a benchmark for readiness; each product is slightly different but when your over-all scores are displayed you will get a readiness indicator; some use green, yellow, and red indicators, others give you a percentile indicator. Whatever the product uses, trust it. These products have excellent validity and reliability and unless you just tank with anxiety on test day, taking NCLEX when the product indicates you are ready will assure your success.

The product will give you an overall score for each Client Needs Category. Review those results. If you have a Client Needs Category below benchmark, create practice tests with questions just from that category. Continue working on that content area until you are above the benchmark.

This is how you can overcome "Hope is not a plan" and progress from practice to testing when you know you are ready, not when you hope you've done enough.

13.3.1 Is It Time for a Test Analysis?

If your practice test scores are not improving (as described in "Monitor practice test scores" above), decipher why by doing a test analysis.

You may have done test analysis in nursing school. After you have completed a practice test review your results and write down the number (# column) of questions you missed for each error type in the Error Analysis Table 13.4.

When you see the number of questions you missed in each error type, you know how to proceed. Let's review how to address each error type.

Table 13.3 Positive attitude mindset

Replace	With
"I hope I pass"	"When I pass"
"What if I fail"	"I won't take NCLEX until I am ready to pass"
"NCLEX is so hard"	"I can learn when I need to pass NCLEX"

Table 13.4 Error analysis

Error type	#
Knowledge gap (did not know content)	
Analysis error (knew content, knew what question was asking, but did not get to the correct response)	
Reading error (knew content but misread what question was asking or overlooked a keyword)	
Focus error (knew content, knew what question was asking, but a squirrel outside the window caught my attention)	

13.3.2 Addressing Knowledge Gaps

If knowledge gaps comprise the majority of missed questions you need to focus on filling those in. Do this by improving your test remediation.

After you complete a practice test, review each question on the test to help you identify content to teach yourself. Review the content, not the question. You want to learn it well enough that you won't incorrectly answer any other questions on that content.

Focus here on the NCLEX "need to know" content. This is the content you have seen in your NCLEX practice.

Use active learning strategies to be sure you learn and understand content. Reviewing a question's rationale, saying "oh, right, that makes sense" and moving on to the next question is not going to solidify your learning. Do not rely on this for filling in your knowledge gaps. Follow these steps for addressing knowledge gaps.

- **Learn, don't memorize, the content**

Use critical thinking in this process of teaching yourself the content that is your knowledge gaps. You can't memorize it from a question; you will not see that same question on NCLEX, you will see the content.

What is going to show up here are the content gaps you brought with you through nursing school. You can't overlook them (remember the CAT testing format—it will find your weak areas!). You need to use critical thinking and brain-based learning strategies to learn and understand the content.

- **Handwrite study notes**

Handwriting your study notes is the most important **active learning strategy** for NCLEX success. When you write notes by hand, you activate learning pathways in your brain that support both memory and recall. These pathways are not activated by typing or cutting and pasting on a computer.

The notes should be **in your own words**. This is not to avoid plagiarism, these are, after all, your own private study notes. Writing notes in your own words forces you to translate the information from what you have read to a higher level of understanding, which supports brain-based learning.

- **Use active learning study notes**

Write study notes and organize them in a way that supports your ability to quiz yourself on your learning. The best strategy is to use loose leaf notebook pages in a three-ring binder.

Draw a vertical line to divide loose leaf notebook pages in half. Each page will have a left column and a right column.

When you identify content that is a knowledge gap, name the content in the left column, then use active learning strategies to learn the content.

This is like using flash cards with a cue on the front and an answer on the back. You are writing your cue in the left column. You can write the cue as a question, or as a statement. Here's an example of study note for HbA1C in each format (Fig. 13.1):

Fig. 13.1 Study notes formats

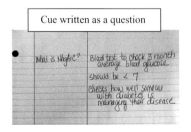
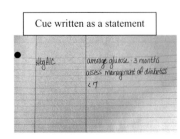

Write your understanding of the content in the right column. The study note is **your** understanding of the content. Don't copy something you've read.

Organize your study binder. If you are beginning with substantial knowledge gaps that you will be filling in with content review, you may want to organize your binder into those review sections such as Fundamentals, Pediatrics, etc. If you don't have major topics to review, you can write your study notes after each practice test.

- **Quiz yourself on your study notes**

The repetition of reviewing your study notes and retrieving the information supports brain-based learning.

This is why dividing the page and writing study notes in this recommended format will help you. When you read notes you have written, you are repeating your exposure. However, covering the right side of the page (the answer) and retrieving the information forces you to retrieve information from your memory, enhancing your brain's ability to integrate and retain the content.

13.3.3 Addressing Analysis Errors

Regardless of the proportion of missed questions in this column, decipher your analysis errors. Is there a pattern? Do you miss ABC questions? Do you forget to apply Maslow when analyzing question responses? Are they in psychosocial questions? If you see a pattern, use the strategies listed above to address those content gaps.

Most analysis errors are really knowledge gaps. You were back and forth between two responses and picked the wrong one. This most often occurs when you understand the "gist" or big picture of the content but weren't able to discern the details that differentiated the correct answer from the distractor.

Address this by using the strategy for addressing knowledge gaps and you will see your analysis errors decrease.

Several prep products provide NCLEX question analysis tools. Some students find these analysis tools helpful while others find them confusing. This is an area where you have to use what works for you.

13.3.4 Addressing Reading Errors

Reading errors are an absolute "no no" in NCLEX questions. A reading error on a passing level question will drop you below the passing benchmark and you will be working harder to get back up above passing instead of staying at or above passing level throughout your exam. This five-step method for addressing reading errors is also outlined in Chap. 8, as it is an effective way to slow down when you are taking a test to reduce test anxiety.

- **Step 1: Read the question carefully**
  Focus on what the question is specifically asking. Identify keywords that focus your attention on what is being asked and provide cues to what the answer might be. If it is an NGN Case Study question, read everything in each tab. Don't read the answers yet!
- **Step 2: Analyze the question.**
  Here is where you are using your critical thinking. Don't read the answers yet! Review what the question is asking; What nursing concept is being tested? What relevant nursing priorities should be considered? What cues are provided in the question? If it is an NGN Case Study, look for the "cues," which are assessment findings and other keywords in the case study.
- **Step 3: Read each answer option**
  As you carefully read each answer option one at a time, consider for each a yes/no/maybe. Even if you read an answer you choose at "yes" don't select it until you have read every answer option.
  If you have any other combination, two answers you selected yes, or maybe, or several have more than one maybe, go back to **Step 1**.
    Reread the question and look for keywords. Did you overlook a keyword in the question?
    Reread each answer. Did you overlook a keyword in the answer response?

- **Step 4: Select your answer** If this is a question in which you simply do not know the content (this will happen on NCLEX as the CAT will deliver more and more difficult questions until you get one you can't answer) then make your best selection and move on.
- **Step 5: Move to the next question**
  Don't change your answer unless you are certain. Your first instinct is more likely to be the correct answer than a second guess. If you are uncertain of an answer and are permitted to go back over questions, flag it for review after you have completed the exam.

Follow these steps in all of your practice testing so this method becomes your habit. If you do get mild jitters on your NCLEX test day, they won't cause you to rush and miss questions because you have developed this as your test taking routine.

13.3.5 Addressing Focus Errors

Focus is an ongoing challenge because everything in our day-to-day lives hijacks our ability to focus.

Your brain is constantly processing multiple short bits of information that come at breakneck speed in 3 s sound bites. Now you must sit and focus for 2–3 h; how can you make that transition?

In Chap. 4 you will find recommendations for relaxing your mind. If you are losing focus in your practice tests, you are going to have to commit to making changes to improve your focus.

When you learn how to practice with focus, you will be better able to focus throughout your NCLEX exam. Just like you can't be successful in a marathon if you only practice 100 meter sprint races, you can't do your NCLEX retest prep testing in short sessions and expect your brain to keep focused for several hours during NCLEX.

If you have an attention disorder, do all of your practice testing when you have followed your routine for managing the disorder. Your practice test scores will inform your readiness. If you have below benchmark scores but say "well, I took that when I wasn't on my medicine" you aren't able to discern how much of a factor that was.

Look for patterns in your focus errors. Do you have more at the end of a long test? If so, at intervals throughout the last half of the test take breaks to refocus your attention. Do you have several missed questions after a difficult question got you off track? If so, recognize the need to refocus and not let a difficult question derail your concentration.

13.4 Know When You Are Ready to Take NCLEX

Your NCLEX test date should be based on your readiness, not on a deadline. If a job you accepted requires you to pass by a certain date, you will want to plan your preparation accordingly. Self-assessment 13.1 will help you know when you are ready.

Self-Assessment 13.1: NCLEX Readiness
Complete Table 13.5 Self-Assessment Checklist to evaluate your readiness for NCLEX. Be honest in your assessment—this tool is designed to help you identify areas that may need additional attention before testing.

When you have checked "yes" for each item on the Self-Assessment Checklist you are ready to take NCLEX and be successful. Your confidence, built through your demonstrated readiness, will help you manage test day anxiety and contribute to your success. If you have your test date set and your Self-Assessment reflects you are not ready, move your test date to give yourself more time to prepare.

Ideally you will not have a long wait between being "ready" and being able to test. If you do, schedule practice tests once or twice a week to keep you "in shape" and do not stress about studying every day.

13.4 Know When You Are Ready to Take NCLEX

Table 13.5 Self-assessment checklist

Administrative preparation	Yes	No
Required documents submitted		
ATT received		
Pearson Vue account established		
Testing center location confirmed		
Testing accommodations arranged		
Knowledge base	Yes	No
Content gaps identified through practice tests have been addressed		
Able to apply nursing concepts across different clinical scenarios		
Comfortable with all NGN question types		
Maintain and review study notes for weak areas		
Test-taking strategy	Yes	No
Consistently using effective question analysis approach (apply critical thinking)		
Demonstrating effective time management during practice tests (not rushing through questions, not overthinking questions)		
Successfully managing stress		
Successfully managing anxiety		
Maintaining positive self-talk		
Reading errors eliminated		
Feeling confident in ability to pass		
Practice test performance	Yes	No
Managing focus during long testing sessions		
Completed test analysis to identify reading, focus errors		
Scoring above passing benchmark on at least six consecutive full length practice tests		
Meeting passing standard on at least on practice computer adaptive test (CAT)		
Meeting benchmark across all client needs categories		
Overall prediction for readiness in NCLEX prep product shows high likelihood to pass		

13.4.1 Final Tips for NCLEX Success

In the days leading up to your exam, concentrate on staying positive. You have done the work and can carry the confidence in your ability to pass into your exam. You don't need to continue doing long practice tests. You have solidified your content. Short practice sessions activate the neural pathways that integrate your knowledge base.

The day before your exam, keep your schedule light and relaxing with time for rest and self-care. Most NCLEX tutors and coaches recommend not studying or doing test practice the day before your exam.

If at all possible, avoid a long shift of work on this day and under no circumstances should you night shift before your test. This is a day for you to get yourself in the right mindset for your test. Do something you enjoy that relaxes your mind and distracts you from worry. If studying helps you feel better, it's okay to look over a few things but don't overstudy.

Keep your mindset in the right place.

Gather everything you need for the exam and have things arranged and ready. Have your ID. If you will drive to the test center, make sure your car is filled with gas. Plan your route and timing for the route.

Also, as part of your preparation, plan to eat a healthy breakfast that includes protein, fat, and carbohydrates. If your test time is in the afternoon, pay particular attention to eating healthy before you begin so you do not experience a drop in your blood glucose during your test.

Exam Day—Follow these tips

1. **Arrive early**

If you will be driving a long distance, consider going the day before and staying in the area, or allowing yourself ample time to

(continued)

arrive early. You don't want a traffic jam or a flat tire to derail all of your NCLEX prep.

2. Center yourself before you begin

Use whatever mind relaxing practice has worked for you to ward off anxiety at your starting point.

Consider a mantra to begin and refocus as you proceed. Suggestions include:

"I am smart enough to be here."
"I did the work and I am ready."
"I will leave here today as an RN."

3. Address your focus set points

If you begin noticing negative thoughts or distractions that result in loss of focus during testing use your STOP method to restore both your positive self-talk and your focus.

You will know your distraction points from analyzing your test results in your practice and you will know your STOP method from practicing it when you took your NCLEX QBank practice tests. This is the rationale for you to commit to practice testing with a full set of questions in one sitting with no distractions, analysis of your test results, and practice using your refocus strategies to determine what works before the day of your NCLEX exam.

4. Don't panic when you see difficult questions

The CAT test will deliver questions up to, and then above, your ability to answer correctly. For this reason, you will expect to see hard questions with content that is not familiar to you. Don't let any of these questions make you lose your confidence. You have done your prep and if you get a question that includes content you are not familiar with, instead of saying "oh my goodness I don't know this" give a chuckle to your-

self and say "this would be the upper limit of what I know."

5. Don't panic if your exam goes beyond 85 questions

If you go beyond 85 questions on your test, remind yourself, with the CAT format, if you are taking questions you are passing. You can pass when the exam ends at 150 questions. But if you panic and lose focus, you risk missing passing level questions and not passing. If you need to, take a break and refocus.

Systematic NCLEX preparation that follows the guidelines in this chapter is the best way to assure your NCLEX success. The preparation builds your confidence, which improves your ability to succeed.

If you will be driving a long distance, consider going the day before and staying in the area, or allowing yourself ample time to arrive early. You don't want a traffic jam or a flat tire to derail all of your NCLEX prep.

13.5 Conclusion

Preparing for the NCLEX after graduation requires dedication, effective strategies, and a positive mindset. By following the practical strategies outlined in this chapter and consistently working to improve your knowledge and test-taking skills, you'll be well-prepared to pass the NCLEX and begin your nursing career with confidence.

When you pass NCLEX and begin your nursing career, the skills and mindset you've developed throughout nursing school and during your NCLEX preparation will serve as a strong foundation for your transition to practice. In the final chapter, we'll explore how to navigate the challenges of being a new nurse, building on the critical thinking, resilience, and growth mindset you've cultivated. You'll learn strategies for continuing your professional development, finding mentorship, and applying your skills in real-world nursing situations.

References

Claudette, M. F. (2014). Lived experiences of failure on the national council licensure examination – registered nurse (NCLEX-RN): Perceptions of registered nurses. *International Journal of Nursing Education, 6*(1), 10–14. https://doi.org/10.5958/j.0974-9357.6.1.003

Kasprovich, T., & VandeVusse, L. (2018). Registered nurses' experiences of passing the NCLEX-RN after more than one attempt. *Journal of Nursing Education, 57*(10), 590–597. https://doi.org/10.3928/01484834-20180921-04

NCSBN. (2025). *NCLEX pass rates.* Retrieved 12 Mar 2025 from https://www.ncsbn.org/exams/exam-statistics-and-publications/nclex-pass-rates.page

Poorman, S. G., & Webb, C. A. (2000). Preparing to retake the NCLEX-RN: The experience of graduates who fail. *Nurse Educator, 25*(4), 175–180.

Part IV

Transition to Nursing Practice

From Nursing Student to Nurse: Transitioning to Nursing Practice

14

Let us never consider ourselves finished nurses. We must be learning all of our lives.

—*Florence Nightingale*

14.1 Introduction

Beginning your role as a professional nurse is an exciting and challenging time. Your success in the transition will depend on your ability to use critical thinking and embrace your growth mindset to adapt to the challenges newly licensed nurses face in their first year of practice. This chapter will guide you in building a solid foundation for your practice, helping you manage the demands of your new role, embrace lifelong learning, and thrive in your nursing career.

▶ **By the end of this chapter you will be able to:**
1. Understand the progression from novice to expert nurse as it relates to your first year in nursing practice.
2. Demonstrate professionalism in nursing practice.
3. Build resilience through effective coping strategies.
4. Maintain work–life balance during your transition.
5. Develop mentoring relationships that support your growth.
6. Embrace your professional identity as a nurse.

14.2 Your Transition to Professional Practice

The transition from nursing student to practicing nurse comes with both opportunities and challenges. This is not new; prior to Covid, about 18% of new nurses changed jobs within the first year with factors such as hospital characteristics, work environment, and location playing significant roles in nurses' decisions to leave the profession (Blegen et al., 2017). You probably can use your critical thinking to predict what has happened since Covid; nurse turnover rate has gotten higher (Calleja et al., 2024). Recent studies show that up to 30% of new nurses leave their first job within a year (Cadavero et al., 2024). This underscores the challenges new nurses face, including steep learning curves, and high-stress environments (Cadavero et al., 2024).

Many health care organizations recognize these challenges and have implemented structured orientation programs and support systems. In Chap. 10, you learned about new nurse residency programs, which have been linked to greater job satisfaction and lower turnover rates among new nurses (Brown et al., 2024).

© The Author(s), under exclusive license to Springer Nature Switzerland AG 2025
C. Thompson, *Nursing School, NCLEX and Career Transition Success*,
https://doi.org/10.1007/978-3-031-85538-2_14

You will want to keep this in mind as you embark on your new nurse transition. Do not underestimate what you are taking on. The better prepared you are; knowing what to expect and using positive strategies to offset the challenges of this transition, the more likely you will be to come out of your first year loving nursing for a lifetime career. Read on!

14.2.1 From Novice to Expert

14.2.1.1 From Novice to Expert: Know What to Expect

In nursing school, you learned to think like a nurse and apply clinical judgment to client care under the watchful eye of your nursing faculty and nurse preceptors. You were able to develop your skills using critical thinking as a foundation for clinical decision making and clinical judgment.

Your success on NCLEX confirms your ability to make safe and effective nursing care decisions in clinical scenarios that entry-level nurses might encounter. However, this foundational knowledge and NCLEX success don't automatically translate into expertise in nursing practice. Research shows that the transition from student to practicing nurse requires time and structured support (Kavanagh, 2021).

Dr. Patricia Benner's influential work (1982) provides a framework for understanding this transition. Her research identified distinct stages that nurses move through as they develop from novice to expert practitioners. This understanding has guided transition support programs ever since it was first published. While you learned in Chap. 10 how this model helps inform your job search, here we'll explore how it frames your journey as a beginning nurse.

As you start your nursing practice, expect to begin as a novice. Although your nursing school clinical experiences were valuable, you haven't yet made independent clinical judgments without supervision. Approach your transition with a growth mindset for learning. During orientation and your work with nurse preceptors, you'll likely have moments—even days—when you feel overwhelmed and question whether you learned anything in nursing school. These feelings are a normal part of your learning journey when you begin as a novice nurse. Rather than letting them discourage you, recognize them as signs that you're growing in your practice.

Understanding this progression helps you appreciate why the transition takes time. Plan to dedicate your first year to learning your role as a practicing nurse, knowing that this investment in your development will build the foundation for your nursing career.

14.2.2 Short-Term Planning

With the understanding that your first months will require complete attention to your transition from student nurse to practicing nurse, make your short-term plans accordingly.

14.2.2.1 NCLEX Preparation

If your State Board of Nursing permits you to begin practicing with a temporary "Graduate Nurse GN" license you will have the opportunity to be hired into a full-time role before you take your NCLEX exam. Tempting as this may be; after all, you've waited a long time for this but be cautious. As you learned in Chap. 13, you do need to devote time to NCLEX prep. Use your critical thinking to make the decision about what is best for you. If you struggled with test taking and test anxiety all during nursing school, you will want to devote your full time and attention to preparing for NCLEX. On the other hand, if you scored well on your end of program NCLEX readiness tests and don't have knowledge gaps to address, you might be able to balance working full time as a GN while you prepare.

14.2.2.2 Life Decisions

Your transition from student nurse to practicing RN (or LPN) is an exciting time and a major life change. It is well documented that both positive and negative life experiences bring stress (Burks & Martin, 1985; Updegraff & Taylor, 2021).

14.2 Your Transition to Professional Practice

Give yourself permission to focus primarily on your new nursing role for the first year. While life events like marriage or moving may be unavoidable, try to minimize additional major life changes that you can control. Your successful transition to nursing practice deserves to be your primary focus during this critical period.

If at all possible, try not to take on other major life transitions in this transition to nursing practice.

14.2.2.3 Continuing Your Education

If you've graduated with an Associate's Degree and will return to school to complete your BSN, consider waiting until you have completed your orientation or nurse residency period before taking on more coursework. If you've graduated with a Bachelor's Degree (BSN) and want to pursue a graduate degree such as NP or CRNA, it is best to give yourself at least one before going back to school.

14.2.3 Transitioning for the Long Term

Your orientation program may include information about ways for you to ease the stress of your transition and enhance your well-being. If that is the case, you may learn about some of these practical strategies in that program. Following these strategies will help you, not just in your first year when you are transitioning to nursing practice, but throughout your nursing career.

14.2.4 Maintain Your Critical Thinking and Growth Mindset

Your learning throughout this book has centered around understanding the importance of thinking critically, applying your learning to nurses' thinking, and embracing challenges as opportunities for learning (growth mindset) rather than tasks to be completed (fixed mindset).

In Chap. 3, you learned about how embracing a growth mindset enhances your capacity for learning and performance. Your transition to

nursing practice is not unlike your learning in nursing school. It will be filled with challenges as you navigate your learning journey. Refer to the practical strategies in Chap. 3 for embracing challenges, setting incremental learning goals, embracing the power of "not yet" and reflecting on your learning.

This foundation hopefully contributed to your nursing school success; let it carry you to your career success. Your ability to use critical thinking to support your clinical decision making and clinical judgment is pivotal to providing safe client care (Schuelke & Barnason, 2017).

> **Clinical Application: Critical Thinking in Practice**
>
> The following scenario demonstrates how two nurses could approach a client care situation. The client is a 69-year-old woman who was admitted to the medical/surgical unit with a diagnosis of community acquired pneumonia. The provider has ordered Ceftriaxone 1 g in 100 mL Normal Saline IV q24 h. The preceptor has delegated the administration of the IV to the new nurse. Let's look at how two nurses approaches to this delegated assignment.
>
> Jay approaches his nursing with a fixed, task-oriented mindset. He verifies the order, checks the five rights, primes the tubing, and starts the infusion according to protocol. While his technique is correct, this approach doesn't connect the intervention to the client's overall condition or her broader nursing knowledge.
>
> With a critical thinking mindset, another nurse, Mara, will do more. *Before* starting the IV antibiotics, she will:
>
> - Review the client's chart to understand that this is community-acquired pneumonia likely caused by *Streptococcus pneumoniae*, which is why a broad-spectrum cephalosporin was chosen.
> - Check recent lab values, especially renal function and WBC count, knowing

(continued)

these affect both dosing and evaluation of treatment effectiveness.

- Review the latest vital signs (T 101.2 °F, RR 24, SpO2 92% on 2 L O2) and lung sounds (crackles in right lower lobe) to create a baseline for evaluating treatment effectiveness.
- Take time to sit with the client to understand their experience of symptoms (fatigue, productive cough, chest pain with breathing) and concerns about their illness.
- Consider what patient education will be needed about both the antibiotic therapy and pneumonia management.

When you are in clinical care as a new nurse remember that critical thinking transforms routine nursing tasks into opportunities for deeper understanding and better client care. Each client interaction is a chance to connect your nursing knowledge with client needs and to build your clinical expertise while providing more comprehensive care.

As you learned in Chap. 1, critical thinkers are curious, open-minded, and eager to understand the "why" behind their actions. These same characteristics that supported your success in nursing school will enhance your ability to provide safe and effective client care.

Every nursing task, from administering medications to performing wound care to helping a client with mobility, presents an opportunity to engage your critical thinking. When you consistently approach your practice this way—asking "why," seeking to understand underlying connections, staying curious about your clients' conditions, and reflecting on your care—critical thinking becomes your natural way of practicing

nursing. This habit of mind not only improves the quality of care you provide but also accelerates your professional growth and development. As you progress from novice to expert nurse, this foundation of critical thinking will help you develop the clinical judgment and expertise that characterizes excellent nursing care.

14.2.5 Be Professional

While you learned about professional standards in nursing school, now you must integrate these standards into your daily practice without the safety net of instructors and preceptors monitoring your every action. Your professional behavior reflects not just on you but on the nursing profession as a whole. Each interaction—whether with clients, families, colleagues, or other health care professionals—contributes to your reputation as well as to nursing's reputation and the public's trust in our profession.

Professionalism is a broad construct that encompasses how you conduct yourself in your practice setting and when you are not at work. Of course, as the very minimum professionalism requires you to:

- Maintain patient privacy and confidentiality
- Document thoroughly and accurately
- Communicate clearly and respectfully
- Stay within your scope of practice
- Adhere to the nursing code of ethics
- Provide safe and competent nursing care

However, professionalism in nursing goes beyond these basic requirements. As you embark on your nursing career, strive to incorporate the elements of professionalism outlined in Table 14.1.

Let's look at how a new nurse begins to embrace professionalism in practice.

14.2 Your Transition to Professional Practice

Table 14.1 Professionalism in nursing practice

Domain of professionalism	Key elements
Excellence in practice	Striving to exceed minimum standards Seeking to understand the "why" behind actions Taking initiative to improve care Maintaining current knowledge Participating in quality improvement
Communication	Using appropriate channels for concerns Maintaining professional boundaries Contributing constructively to team discussions Demonstrating respect in all interactions Managing conflict professionally
Professional presence	Maintaining appropriate appearance Managing social media responsibly Representing nursing positively Demonstrating accountability Showing up prepared and engaged
Interprofessional collaboration	Working effectively with all team members Respecting other disciplines' roles Contributing to team goals Building positive relationships Supporting colleagues

---

Clinical Application: From Student to Professional

Maria is transitioning into her role as a professional nurse where she is in a new nurse residency program with an assigned mentor, Gavin, who she will work with for her first 6 months.

Before she begins her first day on the job, she thinks about what it means to represent the nursing profession. Reviewing her social media accounts one evening, she reflects on posts from her nursing school days. While none are explicitly inappropriate, some show her in her student nurse uniform making silly faces or include casual comments about her clinical experiences. Though she knows deleting these posts doesn't remove them entirely from the internet, she decides to remove them from her feed as they don't align with the professional image she now wants to project.

Maria learns valuable lessons about professionalism by observing Gavin's interactions. She notices how he maintains a consistently professional demeanor whether communicating with clients, colleagues, or members of the interprofessional team. This becomes particularly evident when she observes him handle a conflict with the pharmacy department.

During a busy shift, there's a delay in receiving a critical medication for one of their clients. Instead of expressing frustration or complaining to colleagues, Gavin approaches the situation systematically and professionally. He first calls the pharmacy directly to understand the cause of the delay. Learning that they're short-staffed and managing multiple urgent requests, he works collaboratively with the pharmacy team to obtain the needed medication.

Maria notes how Gavin's professional approach not only resolved the immediate issue but also strengthened interdepartmental relationships. "That's the kind of nurse I want to be," she thinks, recognizing that professionalism involves not just following rules and procedures, but actively contributing to a culture of respect and collaboration. She also recognizes that this is just one example of professional behavior.

Professionalism in nursing is both a mindset and a practice that extends far beyond following basic requirements or checking boxes on a list of professional behaviors. It's about consistently choosing to represent nursing's highest standards in every interaction, decision, and action you take. As you transition from student to professional nurse, you'll find countless opportunities to demonstrate professionalism—from how you handle challenging situations to how you present yourself both in person and online.

14.2.6 Build Resilience

Resilience is the ability to not just adapt but to learn and thrive in the face of stress and adversity. It is not unique to nurses' and nursing practice. You have observed that some clients bounce back more readily from illness or injury, maintaining a positive outlook despite significant challenges. These were your resilient clients.

The same quality that helps clients overcome health challenges helps nurses thrive in their nursing career. Studies have shown that nurses who demonstrate resilience are better able to manage workplace stress, maintain work–life balance, find satisfaction in their nursing practice, and not leave the profession (Cooper et al., 2020; Hart et al., 2014) even in high stress nursing practice settings like critical care and emergency department nursing (Abu-Alhaija & Gillespie, 2022; Mealer et al., 2012). New nurses who demonstrate resilience are more likely to thrive in transition to practice (Chargualaf et al., 2023; Hughes et al., 2021; Poindexter, 2022).

Resilient nurses share characteristics that you have learned about in this book. They have a growth mindset, viewing challenges as opportunities for growth and reflecting on their learning as an ongoing practice for improvement. They build positive professional and peer support relationships. They practice self-care that includes stress management, healthy nutrition, physical activity, and mind relaxation. And they remain focused on their purpose to be a nurse.

Clinical Application: Resilience in Transition to Practice

Maria is 3 months into her orientation on a medical-surgical unit. Her preceptor, Gavin, is known throughout the unit for his clinical expertise and teaching ability.

Under his guidance, Maria has been steadily gaining confidence in her nursing practice. Gavin excels at providing constructive feedback, creating learning opportunities, and helping Maria understand the "why" behind nursing decisions.

Then one Monday morning, Maria learns that Gavin had an accident over the weekend. Though not seriously injured, an ankle injury means he'll be temporarily reassigned to the Telehealth team for 6 weeks. Maria is paired with a new preceptor, Rosalee, who has never precepted before and seems reluctant to take on this role.

Maria is not happy about this change, but demonstrates resilience by maintaining perspective. She finds gratitude for the strong foundation Gavin helped her build. She identifies other experienced nurses on the unit who can serve as resources to her and uses critical thinking to problem-solve before asking Rosalee questions. She starts each of her shifts with mindfulness, reminding herself that she is on a learning journey, not expected to be proficient in her nursing practice at this point in time. She practices mindful minutes throughout her day when she needs to refocus on herself.

Maria begins journaling to reflect on her learning and record her feelings about the additional challenge that this change in preceptor has added to her transition to practice journey. She realizes this experience will help her in the future, when she becomes a preceptor for new nurses.

Through these actions, Maria demonstrates key characteristics of resilient nurses: adaptability, positive coping, emotional insight, and the ability to maintain supportive relationships. Her practice of gratitude—appreciating both Gavin's initial mentorship and knowing he will return—exemplifies how resilient nurses find positive aspects even in challenging situations.

(continued)

14.2 Your Transition to Professional Practice

By the time Gavin returns to the unit, Maria has not only maintained her progress but has grown from the experience. She has strengthened her support network, developed greater independence in her practice, and learned valuable lessons about adapting to change—all hallmarks of a resilient nurse.

A less resilient new nurse would have approached this change differently, becoming overwhelmed with anxiety about the change, withdrawing from learning opportunities, complaining to coworkers about Rosalee's lack of engagement, and allowing the setback to affect their confidence and performance. Maria rose above all of these behaviors and grew through the experience.

Every challenge in nursing practice, from adjusting to schedule changes to handling difficult situations with clients or colleagues, presents an opportunity to build resilience. When you consistently approach challenges this way—maintaining perspective, seeking support, practicing self-care, and reflecting on your experiences—resilience becomes your natural response to adversity. This way of being not only supports your well-being but also contributes to your professional development. As you progress from novice to expert nurse, this foundation of resilience will help you develop the emotional intelligence and adaptability that characterizes successful nurses.

14.2.7 Lean into Your Purpose

Just like what guided you through difficult moments in nursing school, focusing on the outcome of becoming a nurse, when you are a nurse you will want a guide for your difficult moments. In the busy pace of nursing practice, your sense of purpose can get lost in the shuffle of your days. However, this sense of purpose can be the greatest source of strength during stressful times in your nursing practice. While nursing can be physically and emotionally demanding, it also offers profound moments of meaning that remind us why we chose this profession.

When you visualize nursing practice as a balance between inherent stress and inherent reward, you can understand how the profession's challenges and satisfactions interact. Like a seesaw balanced on the point of stress as depicted in Fig. 14.1 Reward Stress Balance, your experience as a nurse can tip toward feeling overwhelmed or toward feeling fulfilled. The inherent stresses of nursing—difficult situations, emotional demands, busy shifts, complex client needs—can weigh heavily. However, the inherent rewards—meaningful connections, skilled interventions that improve lives, being present for significant moments, supporting healing—provide the counterbalance.

This balance isn't static like you see on the figure. It shifts constantly throughout your nursing practice. There will be moments, or even days, when stress feels heavier. But by consciously recognizing and leaning into nursing's inherent rewards, you can maintain equilibrium. The key is not to eliminate stress—that's simply

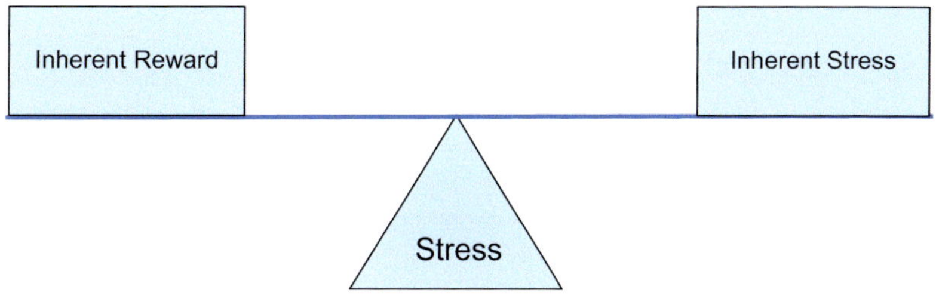

Fig. 14.1 Reward stress balance. (Created by the author)

not possible in nursing. Leaning into your purpose will strengthen the reward side of the balance when you connect with the meaning in your practice.

Clinical Application: Finding Purpose in Difficult Times

For the past three shifts, Maria has been caring for Adola, a 32-year-old mother with terminal cervical cancer. Adola's husband Obasi and their two children aged 4 and 7 have been at her bedside. Adola's condition has steadily declined, and on this shift, it becomes clear that Maria will be caring for Adola in her final hours.

With the guidance of her preceptor Gavin, Maria meets Adola's physical needs with careful attention to detail. She repositions Adola frequently for comfort, provides meticulous oral care to relieve dryness and manages breakthrough pain with medications. Gavin helps Maria recognize the subtle changes in Adola's breathing and circulation that signal her approaching death, guiding Maria in explaining these changes to the family in terms they can understand.

Maria feels the weight of this situation deeply. As a new nurse, this is her first time being primary nurse for a dying client. She finds herself fighting back tears as she watches Adola's children climbing into the bed to lay next to their mother while Obasi holds her hand and prays.

When Adola passes, Maria provides comfort to her family as they stay with Adola. When it is time to provide postmortem care, Maria gently asks Adola's family to step outside, assuring them they can return soon to spend more time with their loved one. Under Gavin's guidance, Maria provides after-death care with the same dignity and respect she showed throughout Adola's care. She bathes Adola's body with gentle, reverent touches, positions her peacefully, and ensures all tubes and lines are removed with care. Maria understands that these final nursing actions are as meaningful for the family as they are important for professional practice. She reflects on this care while she is providing it and finds gratitude for the privilege of being able to be present for Adola and her family during this sacred time.

When her family returns to spend more time with Adola's, Maria listens to their stories about Adola and their family. Even though she herself is heartbroken, she maintains her professional composure while she creates space for their grief. Later, during their post-shift debrief, Maria expresses to Gavin how grateful she is for his mentorship through this challenging experience. His steady guidance helped her provide compassionate end-of-life care while maintaining appropriate professional boundaries. She realizes that having an experienced preceptor who understands both the technical and emotional aspects of nursing has made a profound difference in her ability to support Adola's family through their loss.

Maria finds herself emotionally drained but also deeply moved by the privilege of being present for this sacred moment in this family's life. She realizes that while the technical aspects of nursing are important, it's these profound human connections that give nursing its deepest meaning.

In her reflection journal that evening, Maria writes:

> Today I understood why I became a nurse. While my heart breaks for the patient and family I took care of today, I know I made a difference. I helped them say goodbye. I kept the patient comfortable. I was there when they needed someone to explain what was happening. It was an honor to be present with them during their most difficult moments. Gavin is a role model for how to do it right but I was able to pull from some of my learning in nursing school as well. I am a nurse. It is hard but it feels good.

(continued)

> A nurse who does not lean into the purpose of nursing would tip the balance on the scale and find a situation like this leading to overwhelming stress. This nurse would be likely to distance themselves emotionally from the situation, focusing solely on Adola's physical care while avoiding emotional connection with Obasi and the children. At the end of the shift this nurse will feel overwhelmed by the sadness of the situation and the work of nursing.

Finding meaning in nursing practice doesn't minimize its challenges—rather, it helps put them in perspective. When you feel overwhelmed by the demands of nursing, remember to pause and reconnect with what drew you to this profession. Just as Maria discovered, every nursing experience, even the most difficult ones, offers opportunities to find meaning.

By staying connected to your purpose, you maintain balance between the inherent stresses and inherent rewards of nursing practice. This balance isn't about eliminating stress—it's about strengthening the reward side of the scale through purposeful connection to meaning in your work. When you lean into your purpose as a nurse, you transform difficult moments into opportunities for deeper understanding of nursing's vital role in health care and your unique contribution to your clients' lives.

The same sense of purpose that sustained you through nursing school can carry you through the challenges of nursing practice. Your "why" remains your anchor, helping you maintain equilibrium even during nursing's most demanding moments.

14.2.8 Protect Your Work–Life Balance

The transition to nursing practice brings new opportunities but also new challenges. While you finally have a steady income, you may find yourself facing financial pressures just as you're adapting to the demands of your new role. It's tempting to solve financial stress by picking up extra shifts, especially once you're cleared to work independently. However, protecting your work–life balance during this crucial first year is essential for your long-term success and well-being.

Your first year of nursing practice requires significant emotional and physical energy. Each shift brings new learning experiences, challenging situations, and opportunities for growth. Just as you needed time between study sessions in nursing school to process and integrate your learning, you need time between shifts to reflect on your experiences and recharge.

> **Clinical Application: Protecting Work–Life Balance**
>
> Six months into her nursing practice, Maria faces a new challenge. Her student loan payments have begun, creating more financial pressure than she anticipated. Despite her expectations during nursing school that "when I get a job I will finally have money," she finds her budget tighter than expected with the loan payments.
>
> Maria is becoming more confident in her nursing role, especially now that Gavin has returned as her preceptor after recovering from his ankle injury. Having completed her preceptor orientation period, she's now eligible to pick up extra PRN shifts. The additional income would certainly help with her loan payments.
>
> However, Maria has come to value her time off between shifts. These periods of rest have supported her transition to practice, giving her time to reflect on her learning and recharge for the emotional and physical demands of nursing. She notices that coming back to work well-rested helps her provide better care and improves her ability to remain positive in her learning and adjustment to the demands of her role.
>
> Instead of immediately signing up for extra shifts, Maria decides to prioritize her

(continued)

well-being during this crucial first year of practice. She carefully reviews her budget to find other solutions. She decides to reduce her retirement contribution from 5% to 2.5% temporarily, knowing her loans will be paid off in 10 years. She cuts back on her coffee shop visits, limiting them to work days, and starts packing healthy meals from home rather than purchasing meals in the hospital cafeteria. With other small adjustments she is able to ease the pressure of her loan payments.

Maria commits to giving herself the full year to focus on her transition to practice before considering extra shifts, recognizing that becoming a competent, confident nurse is her most important investment right now.

This balance proves beneficial when Maria faces emotionally challenging situations like caring for Adola and her family. Because she's well-rested and emotionally available, she can provide the compassionate, skilled care her clients deserve while maintaining her own well-being.

As Maria's experience demonstrates, there are often creative solutions to financial pressures that don't require sacrificing the time you need for rest and renewal. Your first priority during this transition year is becoming a competent, confident nurse. This transition is essentially a continuation of your education. This is your priority. While it may be tempting to take on additional commitments like certification courses or extra shifts, remember that this first year lays the foundation for your entire nursing career. Give yourself permission to focus primarily on your transition to practice.

14.2.9 Seek Mentors and Role Models

The transition to nursing practice is enriched by learning from those around you. While your preceptor is your primary mentor during orientation, developing multiple mentoring relationships provides a variety of perspectives and support for your growth. Effective mentors help you navigate not just clinical challenges, but also the professional and emotional aspects of becoming a nurse.

Mentors appear in many forms. Some relationships develop formally through structured programs like nurse residencies, while others evolve naturally through daily interactions. The key is to intentionally seek out and nurture connections with nurses who demonstrate the qualities you aspire to develop. These relationships contribute to your professional growth and help you build a support network that sustains you throughout your career.

Because positive role transition for new nurses has been linked to strong mentor relationships, (Kennedy et al., 2020) you may find that your residency or orientation program assigns both a preceptor for your clinical practice development and a mentor for your professional role development. Take every opportunity to engage with and learn from your mentors.

Mentoring relationships are characterized by mutual respect and trust, open and honest communication, regular interaction, feedback, and growth mindset.

> **Clinical Application: Finding Mentors and Role Models**
> Maria's experience with two different preceptors has taught her valuable lessons about mentoring relationships. The 6 weeks with Rosalee, who was reluctant to precept and provided minimal guidance, helped Maria appreciate the importance of an engaged mentor. Now reunited with Gavin, she consciously observes and reflects on the qualities that make him an effective preceptor and mentor: his clinical expertise, teaching ability, emotional intelligence, and commitment to nursing excellence.

(continued)

"I want to be that kind of nurse," Maria thinks as she watches Gavin demonstrate skill and professionalism and compassion in his nursing interactions. She makes mental notes of how he uses critical thinking to problem-solve, and demonstrates an expert level of nursing practice often guided by intuition as his way of knowing. He gives her reflective feedback and offers encouragement to help her in her role transition.

Maria has also been impressed by Jordan, the unit manager. During particularly busy shifts, Jordan emerges from the office to help with client care, demonstrating that leadership includes being part of the team. Maria notices how Jordan handles conflicts with a calm, solution-focused approach and builds consensus among staff members with different perspectives. When Jordan joins the staff for coffee breaks, Maria makes a point of being present, listening to how Jordan frames challenges as opportunities for improvement.

During new graduate residency sessions, Maria observes her peers carefully. While some spend break time complaining about the challenges of orientation, Maria makes an effort to connect with others who are positive. She connects with those peers when possible for breaks on work days and periodically outside of work hours to share experiences and learn from each other about this process of "becoming a nurse" that they are all engaged in.

The contrast between her experience with Rosalee and her other mentoring relationships has taught Maria the importance of actively seeking and nurturing connections with nurses who demonstrate the qualities she wants to develop. She keeps a section in her reflection journal dedicated to "mentor moments"—documenting specific instances where she has learned valuable lessons from Gavin's and her other role models.

Maria's mentor and role model relationships demonstrate how lessons learned from others can contribute to your professional development. Look for nurses who model clinical excellence and are willing to teach and nurture you as you develop in your role. Be intentional about seeking out mentors and role models. If you are lucky enough to be assigned a mentor, make the most of that professional relationship. In addition, don't neglect the potential for learning you can achieve by looking within your peer group who can also serve as role models and support for your transition from student nurse to professional nurse.

These relationships develop over time through mutual trust and respect. By actively seeking and nurturing these connections early in your career, you create a foundation of support for your professional growth and development.

14.2.10 Develop Your Professional Identity as a Nurse

Your professional identity as a nurse isn't fully formed the day you graduate from nursing school.

In nursing school, your learning about clinical decision making and clinical judgment for nursing care centered around thinking like a nurse. You also learned about what a nurses' role is as a member of the health care team. Basically, your education focused on helping you learn to think and act like a nurse.

As you transition to your role as a nurse, you will also have the opportunity to learn to "feel" like a nurse. This will occur as you watch your mentor and other nursing role models embody what it means to "be a nurse," not just to carry out nursing tasks using expert clinical judgment, but to embody the meaning of "I am a nurse."

Professional identity in nursing is defined by the International Society for Professional Identify in Nursing as "A sense of oneself, and in relation to others, that is influenced by characteristics, norms, and values of the nursing discipline, resulting in an individual thinking, acting, and feeling like a nurse" (KU Medical Center, n.d.). This definition encompasses four key domains:

values and ethics, knowledge, nurse as leader, and professional comportment (Brewington & Godfrey, 2020). Together, these domains describe what it means to move beyond the tasks of nursing care to becoming a nurse as a member of the health care team—one with a unique role that complements the care provided by the team and cannot be replaced by any other member.

Research shows that nurses who embrace professional identity are more likely to thrive in their careers. In a study, 74% of nurses agreed that professional identity is critical to functioning in the nursing role, and 92% agreed that nurses with strong professional identity stand out as having higher impact in their practice (Weybrew et al., 2024).

Let's look at how Maria makes the transition to taking on her professional identity as a nurse.

Clinical Application: Maria's Professional Identify as Nurse

Maria sits at the nurses' station, reviewing her patient assignments for the day. It's been 10 months since she started on the medical-surgical unit, and she's grateful for how far she's come. As she scans the charts, she notices Mrs. Rodriguez, a 65-year-old woman admitted with complications from uncontrolled diabetes, has been assigned to her care.

After receiving report, Maria enters Mrs. Rodriguez's room. "Good morning, I'm Maria, and I'll be your nurse today," she says warmly, making eye contact while updating the whiteboard with her name. Mrs. Rodriguez appears anxious, fidgeting with her blanket.

"The doctor was just in here talking about changing my insulin," Mrs. Rodriguez says. "I don't understand what's happening. Everyone keeps telling me different things."

Maria pulls up a chair and sits at eye level with Mrs. Rodriguez. "I can help you

understand the plan. Would you like to talk about what's concerning you?"

Over the next 15 min, Maria listens as Mrs. Rodriguez shares her fears about managing her diabetes at home. She describes financial struggles that sometimes force her to choose between buying groceries and insulin. Maria notices tears in Mrs. Rodriguez's eyes when she mentions feeling like a burden to her family.

Rather than immediately jumping to tasks or solutions, Maria acknowledges Mrs. Rodriguez's emotions. "It sounds like you're dealing with a lot more than just diabetes management."

Maria collaborates with the health care team throughout the day. She advocates for Mrs. Rodriguez during rounds, ensuring the endocrinologist knows about the financial barriers. She coordinates with the social worker to explore medication assistance programs and connects Mrs. Rodriguez with the diabetes educator.

Later that afternoon, Gavin, Maria's mentor, observes her patient teaching with Mrs. Rodriguez. He notices how Maria doesn't just explain the insulin regimen but takes time to understand Mrs. Rodriguez's daily routine, helping her develop realistic strategies for medication management. At the end of the shift, Gavin tells Maria she did a great job today.

After her shift, Maria decides to write some reflections in her journal.

I can't believe it's been nearly 1 year since I started my job as a nurse. There is much I want to write about at this point to summarize my reflections on this first year, but what stands out to me most is that when I tell people "I am a nurse" I really get what that means. When I introduce myself to my patients and say "My name is Maria, I am your nurse" I get now that this tells them what I will do for them is different than anybody else. And I know this also lets

(continued)

them know they can rely on me to be their point person for their entire journey.

And now, when I meet new people and say "I am a nurse" I see that they get what that means. I don't have a job as a nurse but I am a nurse. Things I learned in nursing school about being professional I see now are a part of me even when I am not at work. I am grateful for all of the role models I have had as I learned this. Gavin has been the best. He is a nurse through and through. I see so many other nurses in my unit and other units who I now see share that bond with me. We are nurses. I have to pinch myself some days.

Of course, I've had so many hard days, but it is finally all coming together. I see myself so differently now than I did last year at this time when I started. I used to think I wanted to move on after a year, go back to school and be a nurse practitioner, but now I am thinking maybe not. I might just stay for a while and savor this special experience that comes with knowing what to do (most of the time) and being my best when I do it.

When you make your transition to nursing practice, you'll discover that becoming a nurse involves more than nursing skills and knowledge. You can look forward to the moment when you realize you have developed your professional identity. When you don't just think like a nurse but you know you are a nurse. This transformation doesn't happen overnight. Just like you will transition from novice to expert in your nursing practice, you will transition to a development of yourself as a professional nurse and member of the most trusted profession!

Your first year of nursing practice, as your journey from nursing student to practicing nurse will give you plenty of ups and downs. Using a growth mindset to accept the learning that will take place will ease the challenges you will face. Using your critical thinking, being resilient, maintaining a healthy work–life bal-

ance, and choosing wisely who you embrace as role models, will help you shape your professional identity. As you begin this journey, remember that each challenge you face is an opportunity for growth, and each experience contributes to your development as a professional nurse.

14.3 Conclusion

Your transition from nursing student to practicing nurse is a significant journey—one that brings both challenges and profound rewards. The strategies you've learned throughout nursing school—critical thinking, reflection, self-care, and maintaining a growth mindset—will serve you well during this transition. Combined with the support of mentors, the wisdom of experienced colleagues, and your own commitment to learning, these tools will help you navigate your journey from novice to expert nurse.

Most importantly, remember that you're not just starting a job—you're beginning a career in a profession that offers limitless opportunities for growth, learning, and making meaningful differences in people's lives. As you develop your professional identity and embrace what it truly means to be a nurse, the foundation you build during this first year will support you throughout your nursing journey.

Welcome to nursing practice. Your adventure begins now.

References

Abu-Alhaija, D. M., & Gillespie, G. L. (2022). Critical clinical events and resilience among emergency nurses in 3 trauma hospital-based emergency departments: A cross-sectional study. *Journal of Emergency Nursing, 48*(5), 525–537. https://doi.org/10.1016/j.jen.2022.05.001

Benner, P. (1982). From novice to expert. *AJN: The American Journal of Nursing, 82*(3), 402–407.

Blegen, M. A., Spector, N., Lynn, M. R., Barnsteiner, J., & Ulrich, B. T. (2017). Newly licensed RN retention: Hospital and nurse characteristics. *JONA: The Journal of Nursing Administration, 47*(10), 508–514. https://doi.org/10.1097/NNA.0000000000000523

Brewington, J., & Godfrey, N. (2020). The professional identity in nursing initiative. *Nursing Education Perspectives, 41*(3), 201. https://doi.org/10.1097/01.NEP.0000000000000667

Brown, J. A., Capper, T., Hegney, D., Donovan, H., Williamson, M., Calleja, P., Solomons, T., & Wilson, S. (2024). Individual and environmental factors that influence longevity of newcomers to nursing and midwifery: A scoping review. *JBI Evidence Synthesis, 22*(5), 753–789. https://doi.org/10.11124/JBIES-22-00367

Burks, N., & Martin, B. (1985). Everyday problems and life change events: Ongoing versus acute sources of stress. *Journal of Human Stress, 11*(1), 27–35.

Cadavero, A. A., Pena, H., Brooks, K., & Kester, K. (2024). Perceptions of new graduate nurses' transition to practice post-pandemic. *Nurse Leader, 22*(3), 312–316. https://doi-org.ezproxy.ycp.edu:8443/10.1016/j.mnl.2023.11.008

Calleja, P., Knight-Davidson, P., McVicar, A., Laker, C., Yu, S., & Roszak-Burton, L. (2024). Gratitude interventions to improve wellbeing and resilience of graduate nurses transitioning to practice: A scoping review. *International Journal of Nursing Studies Advances, 6*, 100188. https://doi.org/10.1016/j.ijnsa.2024.100188

Chargualaf, K. A., Bourgault, A., Torkildson, C., Graham-Clark, C., Nunez, S., Barile, L. T., DelaCruz, F. L., Reeher, D., Eversole, T., Edwards, G., & Nichols, M. (2023). Retaining new graduate nurses: Lessons learned from the COVID-19 pandemic. *Nursing Management, 54*(9), 26–34. https://doi.org/10.1097/nmg.0000000000000049

Cooper, A. L., Brown, J. A., Rees, C. S., & Leslie, G. D. (2020). Nurse resilience: A concept analysis. *International Journal of Mental Health Nursing, 29*(4), 553–575. https://doi.org/10.1111/inm.12721

Hart, P. L., Brannan, J. D., & De Chesnay, M. (2014). Resilience in nurses: An integrative review. *Journal of Nursing Management, 22*(6), 720–734. https://doi.org/10.1111/j.1365-2834.2012.01485.x

Hughes, V., Cologer, S., Swoboda, S., & Rushton, C. (2021). Strengthening internal resources to promote resilience among prelicensure nursing students. *Journal of Professional Nursing, 37*(4), 777–783. https://doi.org/10.1016/j.profnurs.2021.05.008

Kavanagh, J. M. (2021). Crisis in competency: A defining moment in nursing education. *Online Journal of Issues in Nursing, 26*(1). https://doi.org/10.3912/OJIN.Vol26No01Man02

Kennedy, J. A., Jenkins, S. H., Novotny, N. L., Astroth, K. M., & Woith, W. M. (2020). Lessons learned in implementation of an expert nurse mentor program. *Journal for Nurses in Professional Development, 36*(3), 141–145. https://doi.org/10.1097/NND.0000000000000624

KU Medical Center. (n.d.). *What is professional identity in nursing?* Professional Identify in Nursing. Retrieved November 3, 2024 from, https://www.kumc.edu/school-of-nursing/outreach/professional-identity/about/what-is-professional-identity-in-nursing.html

Mealer, M., Jones, J., Newman, J., McFann, K. K., Rothbaum, B., & Moss, M. (2012). The presence of resilience is associated with a healthier psychological profile in intensive care unit (ICU) nurses: Results of a national survey. *International Journal of Nursing Studies, 49*(3), 292–299. https://doi.org/10.1016/j.ijnurstu.2011.09.015

Poindexter, K. (2022). Resilience, well-being, and preparation for the profession: A moral imperative. *Nursing Education Perspectives, 43*(1), 1–2. https://doi.org/10.1097/01.NEP.0000000000000935

Schuelke, S., & Barnason, S. (2017). Interventions used by nurse preceptors to develop critical thinking of new graduate nurses: A systematic review. *Journal for Nurses in Professional Development, 33*(1), E1–E7. https://doi.org/10.1097/NND.0000000000000318

Updegraff, J. A., & Taylor, S. E. (2021). From vulnerability to growth: Positive and negative effects of stressful life events. In *Loss and trauma* (pp. 3–28). Routledge.

Weybrew, K. A., Priddy, K. D., Howard, M. S., & Cusatis Phillips, B. (2024). Building strong foundations: The crucial role of professional identity in nursing excellence. *Oregon State Board of Nursing Sentinel, 43*(2), 6–9.

Printed in the United States
by Baker & Taylor Publisher Services